THE TRUTH ABOUT PHYSICAL FITNESS AND NUTRITION

Robert N. Golden, M.D.
University of Wisconsin–Madison
General Editor

Fred L. Peterson, Ph.D.
University of Texas–Austin
General Editor

John V. Perritano
Principal Author

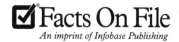

Facts On File
An imprint of Infobase Publishing

The Truth About Physical Fitness and Nutrition

Facts On File, Inc.
An imprint of Infobase Publishing
132 West 31st Street
New York NY 10001

Library of Congress Cataloging-in-Publication Data

Perritano, John.
    The truth about physical fitness and nutrition / Robert N. Golden, general editor, Fred L. Peterson, general editor ; John Perritano, principal author.
        p. cm.
    Includes bibliographical references and index.
    ISBN-13: 978-0-8160-7645-1 (hardcover : alk. paper)
    ISBN-10: 0-8160-7645-6 (hardcover : alk. paper) 1. Physical fitness—Encyclopedias. 2. Nutrition—Encyclopedias. I. Golden, Robert N. II. Peterson, Fred (Fred L.) III. Title.
    RA781.P475 2010
    613.703—dc22

                            2010002346

Facts On File books are available at special discounts when purchased in bulk quantities for businesses, associations, institutions, or sales promotions. Please call our Special Sales Department in New York at (212) 967-8800 or (800) 322-8755.

You can find Facts On File on the World Wide Web at
http://www.factsonfile.com

Excerpts included herewith have been reprinted by permission of the copyright holders; the author has made every effort to contact copyright holders. The publishers will be glad to rectify, in future editions, any errors or omissions brought to their notice.

Text design by David Strelecky
Composition by Mary Susan Ryan-Flynn
Cover printed by Art Print, Taylor, Pa.
Book printed and bound by Maple Press, York, Pa.
Date printed: October 2010
Printed in the United States of America

10 9 8 7 6 5 4 3 2 1

This book is printed on acid-free paper.

CONTENTS

LIST OF ILLUSTRATIONS

PREFACE

The Truth About series—updated and expanded to include 20 volumes—seeks to identify the most pressing health issues and social challenges confronting our nation's youths. Adolescence is the period between the onset of puberty and the attainment of adult roles and responsibilities. Adolescence is also a time of storm, stress, and risk-taking for many young people. During adolescence, a person's health is influenced by biological, psychological, and social factors, all of which interact with one's environment—family, peers, school, and community. It is a time when teenagers experience profound changes.

With the latest available statistics and new insights that have emerged from ongoing research, the Truth About series seeks to help young people build a foundation of information as they face some of the challenges that will affect their health and well-being. These challenges include high-risk behaviors, such as alcohol, tobacco, and other drug use; sexual behaviors that can lead to adolescent pregnancy and sexually transmitted diseases (STDs), such as HIV/AIDS; mental health concerns, such as depression and suicide; learning disorders and disabilities, which are often associated with school failures and school drop-outs; serious family problems, including domestic violence and abuse; and lifestyle factors that increase adolescents' risk for noncommunicable diseases, such as diabetes and cardiovascular disease, among others.

Broader underlying factors also influence adolescent health. These include socioeconomic circumstances, such as poverty, available health care, and the political and social situations in which young people live. Although these factors can negatively affect adolescent health and well-being as well as school performance, many of these negative health outcomes are preventable with the proper knowledge and information.

With prevention in mind, the writers and editors of each topical volume in the Truth About series have tried to provide cutting-edge information that is supported by research and scientific evidence. Vital facts are presented that inform youths about the challenges experienced during adolescence, while special features seek to dispel common myths and misconceptions. Some of the main topics explored include abuse, alcohol, death and dying, divorce, drugs, eating disorders, family life, fear and depression, rape, sexual behavior and unplanned pregnancy, smoking, and violence. All volumes discuss risk-taking behaviors and their consequences, healthy choices, prevention, available treatments, and where to get help.

In this new edition of the series, we also have added eight new titles in areas of increasing significance to today's youths. ADHD, or attention-deficit/hyperactivity disorder, and learning disorders are diagnosed with increasing frequency, and many students have observed or know of classmates who receive treatment for these conditions, even if they have not themselves received this diagnosis. Gambling is gaining currency in our culture, as casinos open and expand in many parts of the country, and the Internet offers easy access for this addictive behavior. Another consequence of our increasingly "online" society, unfortunately, is the presence of online predators. Environmental hazards represent yet another danger, and it is important to provide unbiased information about this topic to our youths. Suicide, which for many years has been a "silent epidemic," is now gaining recognition as a major public health problem throughout the life span, including the teenage and young adult years. We now also offer an overview of illness and disease in a volume that includes the major conditions of particular interest and concern to youths. In addition to illness, however, it is essential to emphasize health and its promotion, and this is especially apparent in the volumes on physical fitness and stress management.

It is our intent that each book serve as an accessible, authoritative resource to which young people can turn for accurate and meaningful answers to their specific questions. The series can help them research particular problems and provide an up-to-date evidence base. It is also designed with parents, teachers, and counselors in mind so that they have a reliable resource that they can share with youths who seek their guidance.

Finally, we have tried to provide unbiased facts rather than subjective opinions. Our goal is to help elevate the health of the public with an emphasis on its most precious component—our youths. As young people face the challenges of an increasingly complex world, we as educators want them to be armed with the most powerful weapon available, knowledge.

Robert N. Golden, M.D.
Fred L. Peterson, Ph.D.
General Editors

HOW TO
USE THIS BOOK

NOTE TO STUDENTS

Knowledge is power. By possessing knowledge you have the ability to make decisions, ask follow-up questions, or know where to go to obtain more information. In the world of health that *is* power! That is the purpose of this book—to provide you with the power you need to obtain unbiased, accurate information and *The Truth About Violence.*

Topics in each volume of The Truth About series are arranged in alphabetical order, from A to Z. Each of these entries defines its topic and explains in detail the particular issue. At the end of most entries are cross-references to related topics. A list of all topics by letter can be found in the table of contents or at the back of the book in the index.

How have these books been compiled? First, the publisher worked with me to identify some of the country's leading authorities on key issues in health education. These individuals were asked to identify some of the major concerns that young people have about such topics. The writers read the literature, spoke with health experts, and incorporated their own life and professional experiences to pull together the most up-to-date information on health issues, particularly those of interest to adolescents and of concern in Healthy People 2010.

Throughout the alphabetical entries, the reader will find sidebars that separate Fact from Fiction. There are Question-and-Answer boxes that attempt to address the most common questions that youths ask about sensitive topics. In addition, readers will find a special feature called "Teens Speak"—case studies of teens with personal stories related to the topic in hand.

This may be one of the most important books you will ever read. Please share it with your friends, families, teachers, and classmates. Remember, you possess the power to control your future. One way to affect your course is through the acquisition of knowledge. Good luck and keep healthy.

NOTE TO LIBRARIANS

This book, along with the rest of The Truth About series, serves as a wonderful resource for young researchers. It contains a variety of facts, case studies, and further readings that the reader can use to help answer questions, formulate new questions, or determine where to go to find more information. Even though the topics may be considered delicate by some, do not be afraid to ask patrons if they have questions. Feel free to direct them to the appropriate sources, but do not press them if you encounter reluctance. The best we can do as educators is to let young people know that we are there when they need us.

Mark J. Kittleson, Ph.D.
Adviser to the First Edition

UNDERSTANDING PHYSICAL FITNESS AND NUTRITION

You have heard this before, but it is worth repeating: You only have one body. You cannot trade it in for a new model. Like a car, if you do not take care of your body with routine maintenance, it will have problems.

Many people are unhappy with their body and are always trying to change the way they look. According to the latest statistics from the Centers for Disease Control (CDC), 33 percent of adult men are obese. The obesity rate is 35.3 percent for adult women and 16.3 percent for children.

Millions of people diet to lose weight. Millions more suffer from low **self-esteem,** many because they are unhappy with their physical appearance. Americans especially put a lot of emphasis on body weight, size, and appearance. We are conditioned at a very young age—by family, peers, and the media—to associate a person's physical characteristics with self-worth. We tend to think of thin, muscular people as individuals who are strong and self-disciplined. We are also conditioned to think that overweight people are lazy and weak.

At school, chances are the most popular kids are good looking and lean. There is a perception, not only in this country but all over the world, that if people are thin and attractive, they will be happy and successful in life. These perceptions have increasingly influenced behavior. Consider some of these statistics compiled by the University of Colorado at Boulder:

■ In 1970, the average age of a girl who started dieting was 14. In 1990, the average age was eight.

■ After viewing pictures of fashion models, 70 percent of the women surveyed became more depressed and angrier than they were before viewing the images.

■ More young girls are afraid of becoming fat than they are of losing their parents or getting cancer.

■ Some 33 percent of women and 25 percent of men are on a diet at any given time.

Yet, being physically fit and healthy is not vain. In fact, it is crucial to a long life without serious problems. Those who are overweight or those who do not exercise regularly often have health problems that can plague them for years. This volume takes an in-depth look at physical fitness and nutrition, the two most important aspects in life. It provides the facts and dispels the myths and rumors about practicing healthy hygiene, achieving fitness, and avoiding some risky behaviors. *The Truth About Physical Fitness and Nutrition* is filled with the data, statistics, charts, and information that will not only give readers the current facts on improving body image but also will help them attain a healthier lifestyle.

Each day we make choices about the foods we eat and the types of exercise, if any, we get. Each choice, good or bad, can harm or help a person's well-being. We might not see the effects of our choices now, but over time, we will be able to reap the rewards or suffer the consequences of our actions.

FOOD CHOICES

The often-repeated expression "You are what you eat" is true. The most important thing we do every day is put food into our bodies. Food is necessary for life. The types of food we consume impact our health in innumerable ways.

Food choices for most people are not generally dictated by health concerns but rather by social and behavioral influences. Most people understand that their eating habits can affect their health. They know that certain foods are very nourishing and provide the body with the essential nutrients it needs to function properly. Still, people tend to fill up on unhealthy foods that can cause a myriad of problems.

What influences peoples' choices? Obviously, people choose foods because they like certain flavors. Most people like foods that are sweet and salty. Others might choose foods that are tangy and spicy. People also eat some foods out of habit. Whether it is a bowl of cereal before school starts or a slice of pizza at the end of the day, most people eat familiar foods. Culture and religion also influence the consumption of food.

Humans are social animals, and meals are social events. It is a way for us to interact with one another. We also eat some foods because they are available, cheap, and convenient. How many times a month do you eat out or have food delivered to your house? People who have little free time are likely to eat food that is quick and easy.

Some people choose "comfort food" as an emotional security blanket. A person might choose to stay home and eat ice cream instead of calling a friend and risking rejection. Some people come home after working late at night and choose to unwind by having a big piece of cake or a huge meal. Many people eat together after funerals as a source of emotional comfort and care. Weddings, where emotions run high, are generally followed by a feast. Holidays, birthdays, and anniversaries are usually celebrated by eating.

Finally, there are also nutritious choices. There are those who eat various foods for the nutritional benefits that healthy food provides.

NUTRITION

The human body is a complex collection of atoms and **molecules**. The actions of the body's various systems, including the circulatory system, depend on nutrients that the body uses as fuel. The body makes some of the nutrients it needs to run, but it cannot make others. It also makes some nutrients in such small quantities that we need to find more of them.

All those nutrients are obtained by eating food. There are six classes of nutrients found in food: carbohydrates, fat, protein, vitamins, minerals, and water. As long as the body receives the right amount of nutrients and energy it needs, the body's cells, molecules, and atoms will work correctly. Tissue will repair itself. Bone will grow, and organs will remain healthy. As teenagers, your body needs different nutrients than an adult or a newborn infant.

Problems arise when we do not get enough of the nutrients we need each day from food. There are many health problems that arise from eating the wrong foods or not eating enough of the right foods. Heart disease, obesity, and growth problems are all associated with poor eating habits. That is why nutritionists recommend eating a balanced diet containing foods from all the major food groups.

Using as many calories as you take in is the crux of maintaining a healthy body. People need calories to survive. Calories are units of energy. When we eat a piece of cake that contains 250 calories, we are really eating 250 units of energy. Weight gain occurs when our caloric intake is more than the calories we expend. The body turns excess calories into fat. Keeping track of how many calories you consume in a day is important in maintaining that delicate balance.

Because each person's food energy intake must equal the amount of energy he or she expends in order to maintain a healthy body weight, the U.S. government publishes a list of guidelines to help people make healthy choices about the food they eat. Based on research and science, the government has outlined its Recommended Dietary Allowances (RDA) as a nutrition standard. The RDA is essentially an amount of selected nutrients that scientists consider adequate to meet the nutritional needs of healthy people. The government has set RDA standards for energy, or calories; carbohydrates; fat; protein; vitamins; and minerals.

To help people understand what the minimum standards are, food manufacturers publish a nutrition facts label on packages of their products. By looking at the label, consumers can judge the nutritional value of a particular food.

EXERCISE

Eating the right foods is just part of maintaining a healthy body. Getting enough exercise is also extremely important. There are two forms of exercise. One is called **aerobic**. Aerobic exercises are high-impact workouts, such as cycling and jogging. Aerobic exercises are performed at a moderate, continuous pace over a long period of time. Aerobic exercises help your body use oxygen more efficiently. Aerobic workouts strengthen especially the lungs and heart.

Strength training, or **anaerobic** exercise, works the body's muscles against extra weight. This resistance training increases the amount of muscle mass in the body by making muscles work harder than they are used to working. In addition to building muscle and toning one's body, strength exercises help the body burn calories, decreasing one's weight.

NUTRITIONAL INFORMATION

Here is an interesting project. Pick a day during the week and keep track of the number of times you come in contact with news about nutrition.

It might be in class. It might be on TV. It might be in talking to your friends or family or reading a story on the Internet or in a newspaper.

Americans are seemingly bombarded with daily news about nutrition. They want to know about the right foods to eat and how to best take care of themselves. People's interest in nutrition fuels an industry that makes billions of dollars a year. Many times, however, what you hear is false. It helps to be educated about nutrition so that you can best determine for yourself if a claim is true or false. However, in many areas, it is hard to distinguish fact from myth. The key is to look at the source and determine whether the person hawking a product or giving nutritional advice is qualified to do so.

When it comes to nutrition, many people turn to their physicians or other health professionals for advice. Your doctor is just one place to go for advice on nutrition. Nutritionists are also experts and have helped many people overcome weight problems by outlining weight and exercise plans.

EATING DISORDERS

Society's focus on the perfect body has led to many problems, especially among women. In the United States alone, an estimated 10 million women and 1 million men suffer from an eating disorder, such as anorexia nervosa or bulimia nervosa. Consider some of these alarming statistics compiled by National Eating Disorders Association in 2006:

- Girls between the ages of 15 and 19 account for 40 percent of the new cases of anorexia diagnosed each year.
- Anorexia increased dramatically from 1935 to 1989 among young women between the ages of 15 and 24.
- The number of bulimia cases diagnosed in 10- to 39-year-old women tripled between 1988 and 1993.
- Of people with anorexia, 33 percent receive mental health treatment.
- Of those suffering from bulimia, 6 percent receive mental health treatment.
- The majority of people with severe eating disorders do not receive adequate medical care.
- In 2005, the National Institutes of Health (NIH) said research funding for eating disorders was only $12

million, while funding for Alzheimer's disease research was $647 million. While 4.5 million suffer from Alzheimer's disease, an estimated 10 million people suffer from eating disorders.

■ More than half of teenage girls and a third of teenage boys skip meals, fast, smoke cigarettes, induce vomiting, and take **laxatives** to lose weight.

■ Of first and third graders, 42 percent say they want to be thin.

■ Of 10 year olds, 81 percent say they are afraid of becoming fat.

■ Of college women, 91 percent say they tried to control their weight through dieting.

Many factors are to blame for eating disorders. Some causes are physical, others are psychological, and others are social. Many people are influenced by what they see on TV, see at the movies, or read in magazines. While the media may not directly cause an eating disorder, the media helps create an environment in which people place an unrealistically high value on the shape of their bodies.

The media, through its advertisements, images, and utter fascination with thin models and celebrities, has caused a toxic environment for many people who are self-conscious about their body image. Studies have shown that magazines for women have more advertisements and articles on weight loss than men's magazines. A 1992 study of 4,294 television commercials concluded that about 25 percent of those commercials had an "attractiveness message." In other words, the commercials told viewers what is or is not attractive. Researchers said that the average teen is bombarded with more than 5,260 "attractiveness messages" each year.

HEALTHY LIVING

Each person has a choice to lead a healthy lifestyle—to eat and exercise properly and to maintain a healthy weight. If a person eats cookies and ice cream and plays video games all day, it is also a choice.

Of course, maintaining a healthy lifestyle is easier said than done. Many things affect each decision. The key to success, however, is to become informed about the rewards and consequences of our actions.

RISKY BUSINESS SELF-TESTS

The topics described in this book should give you a clear understanding of what can happen if you do not take care of your body and live a healthy lifestyle. By being prepared for the choices and challenges that might come your way, you also can understand how to best deal with the risks you might be taking.

Test 1: Health Risks

True or False

The following self-test is designed to help you determine if you are living a healthy lifestyle. To identify whether you might be living a healthy lifestyle, record your answers (true or false) to this short test on a separate sheet of paper.

___I do not exercise regularly.

___I eat a lot of processed food.

___I seldom eat fruits and vegetables.

___I do not play any sports.

___I spend most of my free time playing video games.

___I drink more than one soda a day.

___I consume alcohol.

___I often skip meals.

___When I'm hungry, I reach for a salty bag of chips or a cookie.

___I seldom walk anywhere.

Scoring

Answering *true* to any of these 10 statements means that you are not getting enough exercise or that your diet is poor. It is important that you cut back on your intake of snack foods and increase your exercise level, even if it means doing 20 minutes of housework or walking around the block each day.

Test 2: Assessing Lifestyle Risks

True or False

On a separate sheet of paper, record your answers (true or false) to the following statements.

___I eat breakfast every morning.

___I try to eat a salad and fruits and vegetables several times a week.

___You can often find me playing basketball, riding a bike, skateboarding, or jogging.

___I rarely drink sugary beverages.

___I like to take my dog for a walk.

___I rarely eat fast food.

___I know what the Food Pyramid is.

___I exercise regularly.

___I read the nutrition facts labels on the foods I buy.

___I try to make sure that I eat balanced meals.

Scoring

Answering *true* to any of the above statements means that you have taken steps to minimize the health risks associated with a lack of exercise and a poor diet. Although you are young, you are doing things now that will make you a healthier person later in life.

Test 3: Eating Disorder Awareness

True or False

On a separate piece of paper, record your answers to the following true-or-false test.

___Purging and vomiting are not accepted weight-loss techniques.

___People who suffer from an eating disorder are often depressed.

___People who suffer from an eating disorder will often try to hide their illness.

___Of those suffering from an eating disorder, 90 percent are women.

___Those suffering from an eating disorder will often exercise too much.

___Anorexics have an intense fear of weight gain marked by a distorted body image. They will often deny that they are hungry.

___Many people suffering from an eating disorder will abuse laxatives.

___Bulimics might be prone to **compulsive** spending.

___Bulimics will often have bad teeth.

___A person's **genes** may play a role in an eating disorder.

Scoring

Give yourself one point for each "true" answer and zero points for each "false" answer. Now total your score and compare your score to the maximum:

Maximum Score	Your Score
10	___

If you scored from 8 to 10, that is excellent. You have a keen awareness of the problems facing those with eating disorders. If you scored from 6 to 8, you have a good understanding of the issue. A score of 1 to 5 means that you do not have a grasp of the problems facing those who suffer from an eating disorders and should consult a health professional or ask an adult for advice. Also turn to "Hotlines and Help Sites" at the back of this book.

A-TO-Z ENTRIES

■ ADDITIVES AND PROCESSED FOOD

Chemicals are added to food as nutritional supplements, flavorings, or **preservatives,** and raw foods are altered to promote safety and convenience during consumption. Many people may think that all processed food and additives are unhealthy. However, without these production methods and enhancers, it would be impossible to enjoy tasty foods any time of the year. Also, many of these methods reduce the risk of food-borne illnesses. However, some processed foods and food additives do pose serious health risks.

It was not that long ago that the only foods people ate were those that came directly from local farms. Shipping food great distances was not an option. The food would spoil along the way. People in Maine could not squeeze fresh oranges for juice in January, and it was next to impossible to order a steak from Texas in any of New York City's finest eateries. That all changed when scientists began figuring out ways to preserve food.

The food preservation process was nothing short of a revolution. By processing and adding various substances to food, hectic lives became easier. It is much faster to make a plate of brownies by simply pouring the ingredients out of a box than making the desert from scratch. It is infinitely easier to make instant mashed potatoes then washing, peeling, and mashing boiled potatoes by hand.

PROCESSED FOOD METHODS

Many processed foods have a needed place in your diet. Did you know that milk is a processed food? So too are the frozen vegetables in your freezer. Milk is a processed food because farmers use **pasteurization** to kill **bacteria.** Farmers also **homogenize** milk to keep the fats from separating. Although many people drink "raw" milk straight from the cow, it is safe to say that most people would rather take a sip of creamy white pasteurized milk. Freezing vegetables not only preserves vitamins and minerals, it also makes cooking and eating vegetables convenient and easy, especially when those vegetables are out of season in a particular area. In addition to pasteurizing, freezing, and cooking food, there are several other methods for processing food, including canning, dehydration (drying), and **aseptic** processing.

DANGERS OF PROCESSED FOOD

Some processed foods, such as sugary breakfast cereals, soda, and processed meats, pose health risks. Many processed foods contain **trans fats,** high levels of salt and sugar, and **saturated fats.** Processed meats, such as salami, bologna, ham, sausages, hot dogs, and other packaged lunch meats, can also be harmful. For example, eating huge amounts of processed meats may increase a person's risk of kidney, stomach, and **colorectal** cancer. Processed meats often contain **synthetic** chemicals that are **carcinogens.** A study of 200,000 people by researchers at the University of Hawaii found that those who ate a lot of processed meats had a 67 percent higher risk of pancreatic cancer than those who ate little or no meat products.

Eating processed foods also increases a person's risk for obesity, because processed foods are often high in sugar, fat, and salt. Some scientists believe that eating processed foods high in sugar is an addiction that can lead to weight problems. Dr. Robert Lustig of the University of California in San Francisco reports that processed food laden with sugar can alter the **hormones** in the body and create not only a "toxic environment" but also an "addiction" to food.

According to Lustig's theory, the body steps up its production of insulin when a person eats sugar. Lustig explains that insulin blocks the hormones that control appetite. That process, Lustig says, creates an addiction to food, which is a theory in direct contrast to those who say that people make their own choices about the food they eat.

According to Lustig, food manufacturers should drastically change the ways in which they make their products. He wants them to stop adding sugar to bread, snack chips, and condiments, such as mustard and ketchup. Lustig says processed food is making America fat.

Fact Or Fiction?

You cannot tell what the ingredients are in processed food.

The Facts: Every box, can, and container of processed food, including breads, cereals, desserts, and drinks, have a nutrient facts label on the package. The table not only lists the ingredients in the food but also lists what the additives are and the amount of fat in the food. Consumers can determine for themselves which foods may contain too many harmful additives.

For its part, the Centers for Disease Control and Prevention (CDC) also reports that prepackaged, processed foods contribute to the nation's high obesity rate. Many processed foods are high in trans fats, which can lead to high **cholesterol** and blood pressure, heart disease, type 2 diabetes, and **stroke.** According to the CDC, about two-thirds of American adults are overweight, and about one-third are obese, which is defined as being 20 percent to 25 percent over the ideal body weight for one's height.

Fact Or Fiction?

Most of the salt in our diets comes from processed food.

The Facts: That is correct. Most people get their salt from processed foods as opposed to putting salt on their food themselves. You can check the salt content of a package of food by reading the nutrient facts label on the package. Often, the salt content will vary from brand to brand.

PURPOSES OF FOOD ADDITIVES

What keeps mold from growing on your bread? Why does cake batter rise? You can find the answers in the substances that food manufacturers add to food. Adding substances to food is nothing new. In colonial times, people often used salt to preserve fish and meat; salt prevents the growth of bacteria in food. Generations have pickled vegetables and fruits in vinegar solutions. People used sugar to preserve fruit.

Food additives perform a variety of jobs. Food manufacturers use additives such as **nitrates,** for example, to cure meat. Nitrates reduce the risk of someone getting sick from a food-borne illness such as **salmonella.** Additives also preserve food so it does not spoil during the time it takes to deliver the food to grocery stores and then to your plate. Other additives make foods look and smell better. Manufacturers obviously use these types of additives intentionally.

Other additives find their way indirectly into foods—through harvesting, production, processing, storage, and packaging. For example, tiny bits of plastic or tin from packages might migrate into a food product. Some types of coffee filters, paper plates, and frozen food packages contaminate foods with tiny levels of **dioxin.** Dioxin, which can cause cancer, is created during the papermaking process. However, the traces of dioxin found in food are so miniscule that it poses no health risks.

Hormones also can find their way onto your dinner plate. Farmers often give their livestock hormones to promote the animals' growth. The U.S. government has set limits on the type and amount of hormones allowed in certain foods, such as meat.

WHY ADDITIVES?

There are five main reasons why food processors include additives in their products:

- Maintaining consistency. Additives that scientists call **emulsifiers** give foods a constant texture. Emulsifiers also prevent food from separating.

- Providing nutritional value. Minerals and vitamins are important to good health. Often, people lack specific nutrients in their diets, and nutrients are often lost in the processing of food. Fortifying foods with minerals and vitamins is a good way to reduce **malnutrition** and prevent diseases.

- Preventing illnesses. Various preservatives are added to food to reduce spoilage caused by mold, air, bacteria, and fungi. Some bacteria can cause a variety of food-related sicknesses. For example, **antioxidants** are preservatives that stop oils in baked goods from becoming rotten, or sour to the taste.

- Making food more flavorful and colorful. Some additives make foods taste better, and others make foods look more inviting.

- Helping baked goods rise during baking. When heat combines with some additives, it reacts with baking soda, which in turn causes cakes and other baked goods to rise.

ADDITIVE SAFETY

In the United States, the Food and Drug Administration (FDA) is responsible for keeping a close watch on the additives that food manufacturers put in their products. Before receiving FDA approval, food makers must demonstrate that the additives do what they are supposed to do.

Q & A

Question: What are some natural additives?

Answer: Soybeans and corn are natural additives. Beets are another natural additive. To color food, processors often add beet powder.

DID YOU KNOW?

Common Food Additives

Additive	Found in	Purpose
Algin	Puddings, milkshakes, ice cream	Makes foods creamier and thicker, extends shelf life
Aspartame	Beverages, puddings, yogurt, chewing gum	Substitute for sugar
Butylated Hydroxyanisole (BHA)	Butter, meats, cereals, baked goods, beer, potatoes, chewing gum snack foods, dehydrated	Stops foods from spoiling
Butylated Hydroxytoluene (BHT)	Cereals, shortening, foods high in fats and oils	Keeps foods from changing color, maintains smell and taste
Calcium Carbonate	Some bakery products, frozen desserts, flour	Gives food a nice texture and is also used as a dietary supplement
Citric Acid	Canned fruit juices, cheeses, margarine, salad dressings	Maintains proper acidity
Folic Acid	Breakfast cereals, enriched breads, flour, corn meal, rice, noodles, macaroni, other grain products	Helps prevent heart disease
Iron	Breakfast cereals, enriched breads	Helps enhance diet
Mono- and Diglycerides	Shortening, margarine, baked goods	Keeps ingredients from separating
Monosodium Glutamate (MSG)	Canned vegetables, canned tuna, dressings, many frozen foods	Makes food taste better

(continues)

(continued)

Saccharin	Fruit juice drinks, soda, canned fruits	Substitute for sugar
Sodium Bicarbonate	Baked goods, canned vegetables, cereal flours	Leavening agent; also maintains acid balance in canned products
Vitamin A	Milk and cream, margarine, dairy products	Helps enhance diet
Vitamin B1 (Thiamine)	Macaroni, cereal	Helps enhance diet
Vitamin B2 (Riboflavin)	Cereal flours, baked goods	Helps enhance diet
Vitamin B3 (Niacin)	Cereal flours, enriched bread, macaroni,	Helps enhance diet noodle products
Vitamin C (Ascorbic Acid)	Cereal flours, jellies and preserves, canned mushrooms and artichokes	Preservative; dietary supplement
Vitamin D	Milk, macaroni products, cereal products	Nutritional purposes; prevents rickets

There are hundreds of food additives. The chart lists the most common and shows where they are found and what they are used for.

Source: CNN.com, 2006.

Q & A

Question: What are artificial additives?

Answer: Artificial additives are made by humans. Because artificial additives are made on a large scale, they are cheaper to use than naturally occurring additives.

Q & A

Question: Are natural additives safer than chemical additives?

Answer: Whether an additive is natural or artificial has no bearing on its safety. All foods contain chemicals. For example, ascorbic acid that occurs in an orange is the same as ascorbic acid made in a laboratory.

Q & A

Question: What is a preservative?

Answer: A preservative stops food from spoiling or helps foods, such as cakes and bread, stay soft and fresh for long periods.

In determining whether an additive is safe, the FDA wants to know whether it causes cancer, birth defects, or other health issues. Once approved by the FDA, the agency will write a regulation outlining how food makers are supposed to use the additive.

The FDA also requires that additives not be used to deceive consumers. The government does not want additives to disguise products that are substandard, nor does the government want additives used if they destroy the nutrients in food.

See also: Blood Sugar, Insulin, and Diabetes; Calories and Weight; Obesity

FURTHER READING

Miller, Jeanne. *Food Science (Cool Science).* Minneapolis: Lerner Publications, 2008.

Hayhurst, Chris. *Everything You Need to Know About Food Additives.* (Need to Know Library). New York: Rosen Publishing, 2001.

◾ AEROBIC EXERCISE, TYPES AND BENEFITS OF

Any physical activity a person can sustain over a period at a moderate level, providing a workout for the lungs, heart, and large muscles.

Aerobic means "with oxygen" and refers to how the body uses oxygen in the metabolic, or energy-generating, process. Aerobic exercises involve improving the body's ability to consume oxygen. Whether riding a bike, jogging, skiing, swimming, or skating, aerobic exercise is a sure way to keep fit and promote good health.

Aerobic exercise involves a warm-up period followed by at least 20 minutes of moderate to intensive exercise that involves the body's major muscle groups. During aerobic exercise, the body breaks down **glycogen** to form **glucose**. When done correctly, not only does aerobic exercise maximize the body's ability to use oxygen, it also makes the body's **cardiovascular** and respiratory systems stronger and more efficient. Because aerobic exercise also helps the body reduce fats, it helps tone and shape the body.

AEROBIC V. ANAEROBIC EXERCISE

There are two types of exercise: aerobic and **anaerobic**. Scientists associate anaerobic exercise with power, agility, and strength. Bench pressing weights, tossing a shot put, and sprinting 100 meters are types of anaerobic activities. Such high-intensity, short-duration exercises depend on the body's ability to break down glucose *without* oxygen.

Aerobic activities include, among other things, tennis, aerobic dancing, jumping rope, and swimming. Unlike anaerobic exercise, aerobic activities are done at a moderate, continuous, rhythmic pace. Scientists first coined the term *aerobics* in the late 1960s, when they researched why some muscularly strong people had problems running long-distance races, swimming, or bicycling. Each of those activities requires great amounts of endurance and stamina.

To find the answer, researchers began measuring a person's sustained performance by the body's ability to use oxygen. They found that endurance activities of low intensity and long duration increase oxygen flow throughout the body, thereby increasing stamina and overall health.

AEROBIC CAPACITY

The ability to hike six miles, swim 20 laps in a pool, or run a marathon reflects a person's *aerobic capacity*. Maintaining a high aerobic capacity is critical to a healthy heart and circulatory system.

How does a person maintain his or her aerobic capacity? Aerobic exercise helps promote cardiorespiratory endurance, which is the length of time a person can remain active with an elevated heart rate. In other words, cardiorespiratory endurance is the ability of the lungs, heart,

---

DID YOU KNOW?

Target Heart Rate (HR)

Age	Target HR Zone 50–85%	Average Maximum Heart Rate 100%
15 years	100–170 beats per minute	205 beats per minute
20 years	100–170 beats per minute	200 beats per minute
25 years	98–166 beats per minute	195 beats per minute
30 years	95–162 beats per minute	190 beats per minute
35 years	93–157 beats per minute	185 beats per minute
40 years	90–153 beats per minute	180 beats per minute
45 years	88–149 beats per minute	175 beats per minute
50 years	85–145 beats per minute	170 beats per minute
55 years	83–140 beats per minute	165 beats per minute
60 years	80–136 beats per minute	160 beats per minute
65 years	78–132 beats per minute	155 beats per minute
70 years	75–128 beats per minute	150 beats per minute

According to the American Heart Association, it is important to pace yourself when exercising, especially if you have been inactive for a prolonged period. Your heart rate should stay within 50 to 85 percent of your average maximum heart rate. To find out what your target heart rate is, take your pulse as you exercise. The target heart rate allows you to measure your initial fitness level and then follow your progress as you exercise. To read the table, look for the age category closest to yours, then read across to find your target heart rate.

Source: American Heart Association, 2009.

and blood to sustain intense exercise. Running, walking, and swimming increase the ability of the heart, lungs, and circulatory system to deliver oxygen throughout the body. They also help the body's cells get rid of waste material.

The amount of oxygen traveling through your system increases as you exercise aerobically three to five times a week. The heart becomes stronger and larger and works more efficiently. It does not need as many beats to pump blood through the body.

The lungs also benefit from aerobic exercise. The muscles that control the lungs become stronger. As such, a person's lungs work more efficiently. Those suffering from lung problems, such as **asthma**, respond well to aerobic exercise. The body's circulatory system benefits, too. As the heart pumps more oxygen-rich blood through the body, **arteries** and **veins** become healthier as blood moves more freely.

In short, a person's entire body benefits from aerobic exercise. Not only do the body's muscles and organs become stronger and work better, the body's brain cells also profit from the increase in oxygen. People not only feel better physically, their mental condition also improves from the high-impact workouts. Aerobic activity is demanding, but, over time, a person's body will adapt.

OTHER BENEFITS

In addition to promoting a healthy heart and lungs, aerobic exercises can also help:

- maintain a healthy weight or lose weight. Muscles that use more oxygen can burn fat longer. When your body burns fat, weight loss occurs.

- increase your stamina. Aerobic activity, such as swimming or jogging, might make you tired at first, but, over time, aerobic activity will give you more stamina and reduce fatigue.

- improve your immune system. Your body's immune system fights diseases. Aerobic activity will give your immune system an added boost to fight infections.

- reduce blood pressure and control blood sugar. Aerobic exercise reduces the risk of obesity, heart disease, type 2 diabetes, **stroke,** and certain types of cancer.

- reduce depression. Studies show that regular aerobic exercise can reduce depression. One study, completed by researchers at the Benjamin Franklin Medical Center in Berlin, Germany, studied the effects of aerobic exercise on 12 patients with major episodes of depression that lasted from 12 to 96 weeks. Of those patients, 10 failed to improve when given **antidepressants** for four weeks. Researchers then had their patients walk on a treadmill for 30 minutes a day for 10 days. They found that the exercise caused a drop in depression. Six of the 12 patients demonstrated "substantial" improvements, the researchers reported.

Q & A

Question: What factors affect aerobic training?

Answer: There are three factors that affect aerobic training. The first is the frequency, or how often, you exercise in an aerobic manner. The second factor is the duration, or time spent, exercising. The third factor is the intensity, or how hard your heart is working, during exercise. You can measure the intensity by figuring out the percentage of your maximum heart rate, also known as the target heart rate.

Q & A

Question: How often should I train?

Answer: Most experts agree that you should train between three and five times a week. Each training session should be 20 minutes to 60 minutes long.

Q & A

Question: During aerobic exercise, is my heart rate a good indicator of how hard I am working?

Answer: Yes, it is. As your body demands more energy during exercise, your heart rate increases. As you exercise, your muscles need more oxygen and fuel. Your heart rate must increase to deliver more blood to your muscles to meet their metabolic needs. Metabolism is the chemical process by which cells change food to energy.

Q & A

Question: My sister takes a Pilates class. What is Pilates? Is it an aerobic or anaerobic exercise?

Answer: Pilates is a type of aerobic exercise developed in the 1920s by a German physical therapist named Joseph Pilates. The Pilates method of fitness is designed to strengthen a person's abdominal and back regions while providing for increased flexibility and joint mobility. It also improves strength.

TYPES OF AEROBIC EXERCISE

There are many aerobic exercises. In fact, many of them, including swimming, jogging, and aerobic dance, are fun. Here are some that are popular:

- Indoor cycling and spinning. Forty-five minutes on a stationary bike or in a spinning class can burn 500 **calories** or more. Spinning uses specially designed stationary bikes that mimic the resistance a bike rider would feel if riding up hills or across a flat stretch of road. The first cycling classes you take will be difficult. Start with one or two classes a week, then gradually work your way up to perhaps three or four.

- Jumping rope. Jumping rope is not just a game you played as a kid. Boxers jump rope to keep fit. It is a high-impact, inexpensive workout.

- Jazzercise classes. Jazzercise dance classes are a good form of aerobic exercise because of their intensity.

- Water aerobics. Water aerobics are extremely helpful for people with joint problems, with back pain, and for obese people who want to minimize the stress on their bodies. The goal of water aerobics is to get the heart rate up and keep it there for an hour or more. The water lessens the impact on a person's joints while providing resistance to the muscles.

See also: Calories and Weight; Dieting and Weight Loss; Exercise and Injuries; Obesity

FURTHER READING

Bishop, Jan Galen. *Fitness Through Aerobics.* Upper Saddle River, N.J.: Benjamin Cummings, 2007.

Pryor, Ester, and Minda Kraines. *Keep Moving: Fitness Through Aerobics and Step.* New York: McGraw Hill, 1999.

■ ALLERGIES: DEVELOPMENT, CAUSES, AND TREATMENT OF

Abnormal reactions of the body's immune system to foreign substances known as **allergens.** Everyone, young and old, is at risk of contracting an allergy during his or her lifetime. While allergies can develop at any age, most begin in childhood. Many times, allergies are **genetic** in nature, passed from one generation to another. Health officials estimate that 50 million people in the United States have some type of allergy.

Allergies come in many forms. Some people are allergic to inhaled substances, such as tree pollen, the fine dust from plants and trees. Other people are allergic to foods, such as shellfish, peanuts, and milk from cows. Others suffer from allergic skin reactions brought on by touching or coming into contact with poison ivy, poison oak, and other plants, fabrics, and substances. Some people are also allergic to different drugs. Dust mites and bug bites can also cause allergic reactions.

CAUSES

Here is how an allergy begins. The body's immune system battles foreign **microorganisms** such as **bacteria** and viruses. Sometimes the immune system makes a mistake. It will incorrectly assume that a generally harmless substance is instead harmful to the body. Once the immune system makes that misidentification, it causes the body to produce a special antibody called immunoglobulin E (IgE). IgE protects humans from parasites. IgE, however, does not protect the body from allergens. The IgE antibodies combine with the **mast cells**. Then, when a person again comes in contact with that seemingly harmless substance, the antibody signals the mast cells to release special chemicals called **histamines**. The histamines run to attack the intruding allergen. Histamines, however, cause allergic reactions, such as sneezing, itching, and watery eyes.

COMMON ALLERGIES

People can be allergic to just about anything, especially inhaled substances, such as tree and flower pollen. The most common allergic condition is hay fever *(allergic rhinitis)*. Nearly 30 percent of all Americans suffer from hay fever, and roughly 10,000 children in America miss school each day because they are sick with hay fever. Treating hay fever, is a big business, totaling more than $1 billion a year in the United States.

The symptoms of hay fever—which has nothing to do with hay or fever—include itchy, watery eyes; stuffed up nasal passages; and postnasal drip. Dust mites, animal dander, mold spores, pollen, and fabric fibers can cause hay fever.

Those who suffer from **asthma** also suffer from an allergic reaction. Asthma sufferers have trouble breathing because their bronchial tubes, or air passages, spasm or become inflamed. Symptoms include wheezing, shortness of breath, coughing, and watery eyes.

PEANUT ALLERGIES

Some people are allergic to certain foods, such as peanuts. Peanut allergies are on the rise, particularly in children. Some scientists believe that children are eating peanut butter at an earlier age, which could increase their risks of a peanut allergy. Roughly 12 million people in the United States suffer from food allergies, and 3.3 million are allergic to peanuts.

A recent scientific study suggests there might be some relief for those who suffer from peanut allergies. In 2009, a group of scientists reported that children might be able to stem the effects of their allergic reactions to peanuts by gradually introducing small amounts of the nut into their diets.

Two teams of scientists experimented on 29 children with an average age of five years. All were allergic to peanuts. When the study began, each child received less than 1/1,000th of a peanut per day. That is like splitting a peanut into 1,000 parts. As the study wore on, the children slightly increased the amount of peanuts in their diets. Nine of the children participated in the study for two years. Five of the nine seem to be free of any allergic reaction to peanuts. The five can eat any amount of peanuts with no reaction, the scientists reported. Four others, however, did not do as well.

PET ALLERGIES

If petting dogs makes you sneeze and contact with cats makes your eyes water, you are not alone. Between 15 and 30 percent of Americans who suffer from allergies are allergic to cats and dogs, according to the Asthma and Allergy Foundation of America.

Flaking skin, also known as dander, is one reason why dogs cause people to sneeze. Tree and flower pollen also attaches itself to the coats of dogs. Cats are a different matter, however. An enzyme in cat saliva usually causes allergies in humans. When a cat grooms itself by licking its fur, its saliva dries on its skin and fur, where it waits to be picked up by an unsuspecting person.

If you cannot live without the companionship of a cat or dog, there are steps to mitigate the pet allergies. Vacuum and clean your home often. Bathe your pet often. Have someone else groom your pet in order to minimize your contact with the animal's fur and dander.

Q & A

Question: What is immunotherapy?

Answer: Immunotherapy is treatment of allergies with allergy shots. Allergy shots are usually reserved for the most severe allergic reactions. Generally, people who get allergy shots cannot avoid the allergen, such as dust mites and pollen.

Q & A

Question: Will moving to another state help me get away from my allergies?

Answer: Because most allergies are generally inherited, a person has the genetic tendency to produce the IgE antibodies for many different substances. The chances of one's allergies going away simply by moving to another area are slim. If you move from one location to another, you may just be substituting one set of allergens and symptoms for another set. Sometimes, though, a change could prove beneficial. Before moving, talk with an allergist. In some cases, people who suffer from seasonal allergies, such as those resulting from pollen, might find it prudent to go on vacation to a pollen-free environment.

Q & A

Question: What is the big deal if I do nothing about my allergy?

Answer: Many times, it is not in your best interest to do nothing about your allergy. It is dangerous to ignore the symptoms. For example, you can get asthma and other serious conditions by refusing to treat hay fever. Rashes can spread if they are not properly treated. It is important to detect and treat all allergic reactions.

DIAGNOSIS AND TREATMENT

In treating allergies, doctors often use a skin or blood test called a radioallergosorbent test, or RAST, to determine what a person is allergic to. The skin test involves the doctor injecting or lightly scratching an allergen under the skin of a patient. After a few

DID YOU KNOW?

Common Allergies

Condition	Triggers	Some Symptoms
Asthma	Triggered by a number of things including cigarette smoke, pollen, dust mites, furry animals, cold air, breathing difficulties, changing weather conditions, exercise, and even stress.	Coughing, wheezing, viral infections, tightness in the chest
Hay Fever	Pollen from trees, grasses, or weeds	Stuffy nose; sneezing; runny nose; watery, itchy eyes; eye redness or swelling
Food allergies	Any foods, but most commonly eggs, peanuts, milk, nuts, soy, fish, wheat, peas, and shellfish	Vomiting, diarrhea, hives, breathing difficulties
Eczema (atopic dermatitis)	Contact with pollen, dust mites, furry animals, irritants, sweating	Red, itchy rashes near creases of arms, legs, and neck
Hives	Viral infections, food allergies, and drugs such as penicillin	Itchy, mosquito bite-like red skin; hives may be found on any part of the body.
Contact dermatitis	Contact with a plant substance such as poison ivy or oak, household detergents and cleansers, and chemicals in some cosmetics and perfumes	Itchy, red, raised patches on the skin that might blister

The chart lists some of the many allergens in the environment, some common allergies they trigger, and some symptoms of these allergies.

Source: American Academy of Pediatrics, 2000.

moments, the doctor checks the patient's reaction to the test. The doctor can also administer a blood test to measure the amount of IgE antibodies.

There is no cure for many allergies. However, with the proper treatment, a person can control an allergy. One way to control an allergy is to keep away from whatever makes you sneeze, cry, or itch. Sometimes that is very difficult to do. Drugs may reduce or eliminate allergic symptoms. Some of those drugs include antihistamines, which treat and prevent watery eyes, coughing, and runny noses.

In severe allergy cases, a patient might receive allergy shots. Doctors inject a patient with small amounts of an allergen that, over time, cause the body's immune system to produce less of the antibodies that trigger the allergic reactions.

Sometimes allergic reactions are life threatening. When that happens, a person or doctor must administer a shot of epinephrine. The drug relaxes the muscles in a person's airway, making it easier to breathe.

TEENS SPEAK

Living With Allergies

My name is James, and I love to play baseball and football. But when spring rolls around and I'm out in centerfield, stand clear. I sneeze like nobody's business. It seems I'm allergic to just about everything, including ragweed, pollen, and even my dog, McBeal.

It seems as though I've been allergic to something my entire life. I have been seeing an allergist since I was eight years old. She gives me allergy shots every two to three weeks. I don't like getting allergy shots, but if I want to go out and play, I need them.

Spring is the worst time of the year for me. I live in a rural town with a lot of trees, plants, and flowers. My nose is stuffy when I get up in the morning. I then have a sneezing fit. There is always a box of tissues near my bed. My mother puts plastic coverings on my bed's box spring to stop dust mites and other allergens from sticking to the bed. She washes my sheets and blanket twice a week.

But don't feel sorry for me. My cousin has an allergy that is much worse than mine. Her name is Lisa, and she's two years older than me. Lisa has always been allergic to peanuts. For the most part, she has steered clear of peanuts her whole life. She reads labels to make sure there are no peanut products in her food. The other day she was out with some friends at a Mexican restaurant. She bit into her friend's quesadilla. The next thing she knew, she was in an ambulance on the way to the hospital.

It seemed that inside the quesadilla was walnut pesto. One time Lisa was in Asia with her parents. She had to eat fried chicken all the time to make sure she stayed away from peanut products used in cooking.

Sometimes I get frustrated with my allergies, but I continue on. Hopefully I won't have to get those allergy shots forever.

FURTHER READING

Bowers, Elizabeth Shimer, and Paul M. Ehrlich. *Living with Allergies.* New York: Facts On File, 2008.

Ford, Jean. *Breathe Easy! A Teen's Guide to Allergies and Asthma.* Broomall, Pa.: Mason Crest Publishers, 2005.

Moragne, Wendy. *Allergies* (Twenty-first Century Medical Library). Kirkland, Wash.: 21st Century, 1999.

■ ANOREXIA NERVOSA

Self-imposed starvation accompanied by an irrational fear of gaining weight. Anorexia is a **chronic,** potentially life-threatening mental illness characterized by severe weight loss caused by self-starvation. Although anorexia also effects boys and young men, it is most commonly found in teenage girls and young women. In addition to the intense fear of weight gain, anorexics have a distorted image of their bodies. They often deny that they are hungry. Women will also suffer from **amenorrhea,** the absence of three consecutive menstrual cycles.

The term *anorexia* means "loss of appetite." However, the term does not accurately define the condition. Anorexics often ignore hunger signals as they try to control their desire to eat. Yet, anorexics remain preoccupied with food and often cook for themselves or others.

TWO TYPES

There are two subtypes of anorexia. One type is called *restricting anorexia*. Restricting anorexia is the classic form of the condition, in which people maintain their low body weight by carefully regulating the foods they eat. In some cases, people excessively exercise and starve themselves to get their weight down.

Binging (and purging) is another subtype of anorexia. In these cases, individuals restrict the amount of food they eat by binge eating, or ingesting huge quantities of food at once. After they have binged, these individuals often purge the foods from their system by self-induced vomiting. Others also misuse **laxatives** or **diuretics** or give themselves enemas. Binging and purging become classified as bulimia when the behavior occurs twice a week for three months, not just sporadically.

AT RISK

Young women are more likely to suffer from the condition than young men. Anorexia usually begins in adolescence, although it can develop any at time in a person's life. Between 1 and 2 percent of all young women develop the condition. The number of older women suffering from anorexia is on the rise. Many women from 50 to 70 years of age also develop the illness.

Caucasian woman who are high academic achievers and who have a goal-driven personality or a family that pushes them to achieve goals are the most likely to suffer from anorexia. A survey published in 2007 in the scientific journal *Biological Psychiatry* found that 0.9 percent of women had anorexia at some point in their lives.

Although anorexia is known chiefly as a female illness, doctors have diagnosed males as young as seven years old with the condition. A person with a history of anorexia in his or her family is more likely to develop the condition compared to someone who does not have a family history of the disease.

Researchers have yet to discover what causes anorexia. Most suspect that combinations of **genetic,** biological, social, psychological, and emotional factors are to blame.

Eating disorders, such as anorexia, tend to run in families. An individual with a relative who suffers from anorexia is 10 to 50 times more likely to have an eating disorder compared to someone who does not have a relative suffering from the illness.

Q & A

Question: What should I do if I think someone I know has anorexia?

Answer: According to the U.S. Department of Health and Human Services, if someone you know is showing signs of anorexia, you need to find a time and place to talk with your friend. Make sure it is a quiet place where you will not be disturbed. Tell your friend what is bothering you. Be honest, and explain to your friend that her or his eating or exercising habits might be signs of a problem. Tell your friend it might be wise to talk to a counselor or doctor who knows something about eating habits. If your friend will not admit that she or he has a problem, avoid any conflict. Tell your friend you are always available to talk. Do not blame your friend. Do not be judgmental.

Some researchers say there are biological reasons why some people have an eating disorder. Research shows that a **neurotransmitter** called **serotonin** tamps down a person's desire for food. Neurotransmitters are chemicals that transmit signals between brain cells.

Social and cultural factors also can play a huge role in determining whether someone is anorexic. For example, anorexia is very common in industrialized nations, such as the United States, where thinness is a positive social and cultural trait. Images of the perfect female and male body abound in these cultures. Whether through television, film, magazines, or the Internet, beautiful women and men sell everything from shoes to shampoo. The media reinforce these images. This culture of thinness puts a lot of pressure and stress on some people whose goal is to achieve the "perfect" body. This social and cultural environment may cause, or at the very least reinforce, a tendency toward anorexia. One study found that women's magazines have more articles on diet and weight reduction than magazines read by men. According to the study, the magazines most read by women, ages 18 to 24 had 10 times more information on diet than magazines read by men in the same age group.

Q & A

Question: What percentage of males suffer from eating disorders?

Answer: According to one study, 10 percent of males suffer from an eating disorder. However, women with eating disorders still outnumber men by 15 to one. Some studies show that many young men who suffer from eating disorders are not accurately diagnosed with the disorder, because anorexia is generally associated with girls and women. Most of the research on eating disorders centers on women. However, as many as 1 million men suffer from these afflictions.

Moreover, people who come from overprotective families or families that emphasize overachievement are more likely to have anorexia. In addition, certain professions, such as those of fashion models and certain athletes, emphasize thinness and low body weight. Female athletes are easy targets for anorexia. Team pressure, coaches, and family often encourage female athletes to lose weight to better their performance.

Q & A

Question: Is it possible to have anorexia without losing a lot of weight?

Answer: Yes, someone can have anorexia without weight loss. Children who are still growing are expected to increase their body weight. If they diet during those years and grow taller without gaining weight, they may drop below 85 percent of the healthy body weight for the new height, and, in that case, doctors will often diagnose them with anorexia.

Psychological and emotional factors also play a role, as there are several personality traits that are associated with anorexia. People who are perfectionists or obsessive or who have low **self-esteem** are prone to the illness. Physical or sexual abuse can also trigger anorexia.

SYMPTOMS

The symptoms of anorexia include:

- denying feelings of hunger
- avoiding social gatherings where food is served
- eating in secrecy
- eating foods in a certain order

- excessive chewing
- rearranging food on the plate
- eating unnaturally small amounts of food
- dramatic weight loss
- obsessing with dieting and weight loss
- seeing oneself as overweight when someone clearly is not
- basing self-worth on body weight and body image
- excessive exercise regime

HEALTH EFFECTS

Anorexics can have many health problems. Because they are not getting enough calories or nutrients into their systems, their bodies will slowly shut down, causing severe physical, emotional, and behavioral problems. Those suffering from anorexia can suffer from the following:

- loss of menstrual periods in women
- dry, brittle bones due to a lack of calcium in the body
- lowered resistance to illness
- hair loss
- brittle fingernails and toenails
- bruising
- lack of sleep
- muscle loss and weakness
- fainting
- fatigue
- heart trouble and low blood pressure
- digestive problems
- poor circulation
- anemia
- stunted growth
- death

DEATH AND ANOREXIA

The most frequent causes of death among anorexics are suicide and problems arising from **malnutrition.** Anorexics also suffer from behavioral problems, including depression, feelings of isolation, and difficulty concentrating.

The suicide rate for anorexics is high, totaling half of all anorexic deaths in the United States. Moreover, drug and alcohol abuse among anorexics is high. Some studies report that between 12 and 18 percent of anorexics abuse alcohol or drugs. Heart disease, however, is the most common cause of death.

The health problems of anorexic women are myriad. Anorexia decreases a woman's chance of having a baby. An anorexic pregnant woman faces a high risk of having a miscarriage, having a **Cesarean section,** or delivering an infant with low birth weight or birth defects.

TEENS SPEAK

I Am an Anorexic

My name is Judy, and I suffer from anorexia. Ever since I can remember, I was mentally abused by my mother. She had high expectations of me.

Even though I brought home A's on my report cards, my mother wanted me to be perfect all the time. I worked as hard as I could. I tried to be perfect, but it was impossible. I ran cross-country in school and always came in third or fourth. I tried hard to come in first place, but I just couldn't, no matter how hard I tried. My mother told me I was a loser, that I didn't have the determination to be a winner.

I used to cry myself to sleep at night. All I wanted was for my mother to be proud of me. Even though I was not fat, I began dieting, hoping that I would become a faster runner and that my mother would love me. I would practice every day, running six to seven miles. Sometimes I would do well in a meet, other times not.

It was never enough for my mother. She told me I was worthless, unlovable, ugly, and fat. One time I got a B+ in math. My mother was furious. She told me I was stupid and that she wished that I had not been born.

Although I now know I was none of these things, my mother made me believe I was the most useless, ugliest person on the planet.

To try to regain some control over my life, and to try to reach the unrealistic goal my mother had set, I stopped eating breakfast. Then I stopped eating lunch. I was going to be the most beautiful girl my mother would ever see. I ran, and ran, and ran. Not only did I want a perfect figure—my mother was a beauty queen in college—but I also wanted my mother's love.

I was losing weight. First five pounds. Then six. Then 10. Then 15. It still wasn't enough. My mother didn't even notice. I then started purging. After dinner, I would go into the bathroom or outside and force myself to vomit.

Then one day a good friend of mine, Julia, confronted me. She noticed that I had been losing weight. She knew what my mother was like. She knew my father didn't live with us. "Judith, you're my friend," Julia said. "I care about you. You are losing too much weight. If you don't do something, I'm afraid I'm going to lose my best friend. How can I help you?"

Of course I didn't listen to her at first. Then reality began to sink in. All my clothes were too big on me. My skin was turning pale. Finally, one day after school, I took Julia aside. "Will you help me?" I pleaded, crying into her shoulder.

The next day Julia and I went to see one of our favorite teachers. Soon, I got the help I needed. People did care about me. I was not alone. While in treatment, I went to live with my dad. We have a good life together. I'm going to go to college in the fall. I still talk to my mother. I know that she has her own demons to deal with. Someday things will be okay between the two of us. In the meantime, I'm glad I'm alive.

TREATMENT

There are no drugs to cure anorexia, although some people may benefit from drugs that treat depression. Those who get into treatment early enough, including **psychotherapy,** have a good chance at beating the illness. Studies show that about half of those who seek treatment recover fully.

The first part of treatment, which usually includes hospitalization, is restoring a person's normal body weight. Once doctors reverse the weight loss, they can deal with the physical and psychological aspects of the disorder. With proper treatment, the psychological problems related to anorexia will begin to disappear.

At the center of the treatment is psychotherapy. Anorexics are encouraged to deal with the underlying emotional reasons for the disorder. The therapist often tries to change a patient's unhealthy thoughts and behaviors associated with the illness. Many times, patients find themselves in group therapy with others who suffer from the same affliction. In group therapy, people share their experiences with others. For those living at home, family therapy is also important.

Getting a friend or relative to seek treatment is the first and biggest hurdle that friends and families face. Because most people suffering from anorexia do not believe they have a problem, others need to take action. Sometimes an intervention is necessary. During an intervention, family members and friends, along with a qualified interventionist, confront the person and tell him or her how the illness is impacting their lives. The goal of the intervention is to get the friend or family member into treatment.

If anorexia is left untreated, the consequences can be severe. The condition can cause irreversible damage to a person, including heart and kidney trouble, bone loss, muscle damage, and death. Anorexia nervosa has one of the highest death rates of any mental disorder. From 5 to 20 percent of those who suffer from anorexia will die. Those who undergo treatment often relapse. Almost 30 percent of patients will have problems for their entire lives.

See also: Body Image; Bulimia Nervosa; Eating Disorders: Causes, Symptoms, and Diagnoses of; Nutritional Guidelines and Healthy Diets

FURTHER READING

Augustyn Lawton, Sandra, ed. *Eating Disorders Information for Teens* (Teen Health Series). Detroit: Omnigraphics, 2005.

Hall, Lindsey. *Anorexia Nervosa: A Guide to Recovery.* Carlsbad, Calif.: Gurze Books, 1999.

Petit, Christine. *Empty: A Story of Anorexia*. Grand Rapids, Mich.: Fleming H. Revell, 2006.

■ BLOOD SUGAR, INSULIN, AND DIABETES

Blood sugar, or **glucose,** is the body's main source of energy. **Insulin** is a **hormone** that controls the amount of glucose in the bloodstream. Diabetes is a condition in which the body cannot control the level of glucose in the blood.

Diabetes occurs when the body's system that regulates blood sugar fails because of the lack of insulin. As such, glucose cannot pass into the body's cells to be burned for energy. Glucose instead builds up in the blood, leading to an abnormally high blood glucose level.

The response by the body to high levels of glucose can be devastating as it tries to eliminate excess sugar. The body must then use fat and proteins from the muscles for energy. When that happens, the body's natural process of converting glucose to energy is disrupted.

BLOOD SUGAR

Like a car or a truck, your body needs fuel to move. Your body's fuel comes in the form of glucose, or blood sugar. Have you ever eaten a candy bar and felt a burst of energy afterward? Every time you eat a meal, your body converts carbohydrates to glucose.

Carbohydrates are chemical **compounds** containing carbon, hydrogen, and oxygen. The simplest carbohydrates are sugars, such as glucose and fructose. When you eat, your body's digestive system converts these carbohydrates to glucose. Insulin helps the body process glucose. Your body turns some glucose into energy; it also stores some glucose in the liver and muscles. Your body converts this surplus, or stored, glucose to fat.

When you have too little blood sugar in your system, you have a condition known as **hypoglycemia.** Low blood sugar can cause a variety of problems, including fatigue, forgetfulness, and poor concentration. You might even faint. Many people experience these and other symptoms throughout their lives. The symptoms usually disappear once the body balances out the level of glucose in the bloodstream.

Have you ever felt light-headed just before lunch? What happened after you ate? That symptom went away. After you ate, your body received a rush of sugar that restored your natural glucose level.

A drop in blood sugar is not healthy. It can affect a person's organs and systems. For example, glucose is the main nutrient that the nervous system requires to function properly. The body's nervous system consists of the brain and the spinal cord, and it requires a continuous supply of glucose to work correctly.

Low blood sugar levels also can harm the circulatory system, which pumps blood throughout the body. A drop in blood sugar will often cause your heart to race. You might also have difficulty breathing. Your hands and feet might become cold.

Too much glucose in one's system is not healthy, either. Too much blood sugar causes **hyperglycemia,** mostly the result of overeating. Eating food that is high in sugar also can lead to elevated levels of glucose in the blood stream. Symptoms of hyperglycemia include frequent urination, dry mouth, weight loss, blurred vision, and excessive thirst. If a person's blood sugar level is high for a long period, he or she is at risk of developing complications from diabetes, such as eyesight trouble, kidney damage, and heart disease.

INSULIN

Insulin is a hormone produced by the pancreas that controls how the body converts carbohydrates, proteins, and fats into glucose. High levels of sugar in the bloodstream encourage special cells in the pancreas, called *beta cells,* to produce insulin. The body then uses that insulin to transfer the sugar to the body's cells; the cells use the sugar for energy. Insulin also turns glucose into **glycogen.** Glycogen is stored in the liver and muscle tissue. Your body taps into glycogen and uses it for fuel when glucose levels run low.

DIABETES

About 200 million people around the globe suffer from diabetes. Each year, 20 million are diagnosed with the affliction. There are many factors that cause diabetes. Some are **genetic,** and others relate to one's environment or lifestyle. If left untreated, elevated levels of blood sugar can damage the eyes, kidneys, heart, and feet.

There are two types of diabetes, type 1 and type 2. Type 2 diabetes is the most common. Other types affect only a small portion of people. Pregnant women can suffer from gestational diabetes. Gestational diabetes occurs when a pregnant woman's hormones inhibit her body's ability to produce insulin.

Fact Or Fiction?

Type 2 diabetes is less serious than type 1 diabetes.

The Facts: In many respects, type 2 diabetes is more serious. Why is that? People might have type 2 diabetes for years before they are diagnosed by a doctor. That means they could have already developed long-term complications from the disease without knowing.

Type 1 diabetes was once known as *juvenile-onset diabetes* or *insulin-dependent diabetes.* Type 1 diabetes can appear during childhood or adolescence, although it can form at any age.

With type 1 diabetes, the beta cells in the pancreas have usually been destroyed by the diabetic's immune system. The immune system, which fights disease and infections, mistakes the beta cells for invaders. As such, the immune system attacks the beta cells and kills them off. Because there are no beta cells to produce insulin, the body's blood glucose level rises, depriving the body of necessary fuel. People who suffer from type 1 diabetes often become tired, dehydrated, and extremely thirsty. They will also lose weight.

Fact Or Fiction?

I have diabetes, but I feel well. That means my glucose level is well controlled.

The Facts: You can feel well and still have a high blood sugar level. The best way to find out if your blood sugar is high is to test it regularly.

To make up for the lack of glucose, the body still needs energy. As such, it begins to break down fat and proteins found in muscles. The body then uses that stored glucose as an energy source. When the body starts breaking down stored fats for energy, it can lead to a condition called *diabetic ketoacidosis.* Ketoacidosis is a very serious condition caused by very high blood sugar levels, in which ketones, the acid by-products of fat, increase the blood's acidic level. The result can be deadly.

Fact Or Fiction?

People with diabetes should avoid sugar.

The Facts: Not necessarily. In fact, with all the processed foods at our disposal, it is next to impossible to avoid consuming some sugar. Many nutritious foods, such as fruits, contain natural sugars. You can limit your sugar intake by not adding sugar to food or drink. You should also avoid sugary snacks and beverages.

TYPE 2 DIABETES

Type 2 diabetes was once known as maturity-onset or non–insulin-dependent diabetes. Obesity is the main trigger of type 2 diabetes in teenagers. In type 2 diabetes, the body's cells become resistant to insulin or the pancreas produces minimal amounts of the hormone. Over time, the lack of insulin results in high blood sugar levels. As such, the cells in the body do not receive their fair share of glucose. With limited glucose, cells have reduced energy. In its never-ending quest for

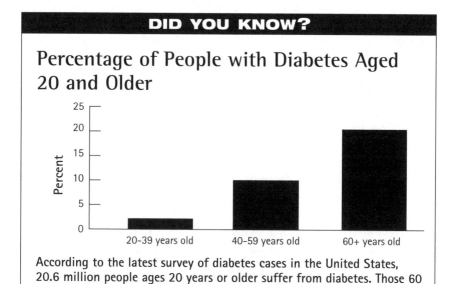

DID YOU KNOW?

Percentage of People with Diabetes Aged 20 and Older

According to the latest survey of diabetes cases in the United States, 20.6 million people ages 20 years or older suffer from diabetes. Those 60 years or older account for 20.9 percent of all people with diabetes. The chart above shows the estimated percentage of cases based on age.

Source: Centers for Disease Control and Prevention, 2005.

energy, the body begins breaking down stored fats. Symptoms of type 2 diabetes include fatigue, increased urination, gradual weight loss, and increased thirst.

TREATING DIABETES

The most important aspect of treating diabetes is looking after oneself. Diabetics must monitor their own blood glucose levels and keep blood sugar levels within the 75–130-milligrams-per-deciliter (mg/dl) range. That means a person must test himself or herself every day and then adjust treatment depending on the results of those blood tests.

What a person eats is just one of the factors that affect blood glucose level. Exercise and taking pills specially made for sufferers of type 2 diabetes also help to control the disease. Insulin injections are another treatment.

Daily exercise helps lower glucose levels. Doctors often prescribe pills that help the body increase the amount of insulin it produces for those who suffer from type 2 diabetes. Some pills slow down the digestion of carbohydrates.

Those who suffer from type 1 diabetes can control their blood sugar levels by insulin injections. Those who suffer from type 2 diabetes may also need insulin injections. If you are diabetic and do not control you blood sugar level, you could experience hypoglycemia or hyperglycemia.

STRIKING A BALANCE

Controlling blood sugar levels and keeping tabs on one's diabetes might seem like a full-time job, especially for a teenager. A diabetic teen just can't grab a snack any time he or she feels like it.

Teenagers who suffer from diabetes are constantly balancing their lives and the disease. For some teens, getting insulin shots every day is not as difficult as planning what to eat at every meal. With a little patience and knowledge, a person can control diabetes. Although everyone should eat a well-balanced diet, such a diet is extremely important to those who suffer from diabetes. Complex carbohydrates are necessary because the body digests them slowly. You can find complex carbs in grains, fruits, and vegetables.

Like diet, exercise is important for everyone, especially those with diabetes. Did you know that two of every three Americans are overweight? As a nation, we eat too many **calories** and too much fat. Exercise affects the body's insulin level. If your blood sugar level is high, exercise is one of the best ways to get it back to a normal level. Physical activity also helps the body burn glucose more efficiently. The more calories you burn, the more food you can eat without gaining weight.

One of the biggest problems for teenage diabetics, however, is psychological. They think they are alone and that no one else knows what they are going through. At the same time, most teens want to fit in. Many fear that their peers will reject them because of their illness. Diabetic teens might feel isolated or have low **self-esteem.** When everyone is eating pizza and hamburgers on a Saturday night after the football game, those suffering from diabetes might feel left out because they cannot indulge in these junk food binges.

Also, because teenagers often experiment with alcohol and drugs, the risks of drug and alcohol abuse are magnified for diabetics. Substance abuse impacts the body's **metabolism,** which is the rate at which the body uses energy. Abusing drugs and alcohol makes it nearly impossible for diabetics to control their blood sugar levels. In addition, because drugs and alcohol impair a person's judgment, those with diabetes are often blind to the changes in their bodies and are therefore less likely to take proper precautions. Diabetics can find a support group by contacting the American Diabetics Association.

See also: Food Groups; Nutritional Guidelines and Healthy Diets

FURTHER READING
Ferber, Elizabeth. *Diabetes.* Brookfield, Conn.: Millbrook Press, 1996.
Walker, Rosemary, and Jill Rodgers. *Diabetes: A Practical Guide to Managing Your Health.* New York: DK Publishing, 2005.

■ BODY IMAGE

A person's perception of his or her physical appearance, which in many cases is radically different from how that person actually appears. A perfectly toned 20-year-old fitness freak with washboard abs might look amazing walking down the street. However, when that person looks in the mirror, what does he see? Does he see a hunk? Does she see a hottie? Interestingly, that person might have a very poor body image.

Body image can affect a person's **self-esteem** and exercise habits. In many cases, poor body image can lead to eating disorders, such as bulimia and anorexia. How you view your own body can also affect your relationships with other people. In teenagers, there is a direct connection between body image and self-worth. Teens often care deeply about how others see them.

CULTURAL INFLUENCES

What do you see when *you* look in the mirror? Do you see someone whose nose is too big, or just right? Do you see someone whose legs are pudgy, or someone whose legs are strong and healthy? The answers to these questions will give you a good indication of how you view your body.

Body image plays a big role in the psyche of all Americans, and a lot of Americans are unhappy with their bodies. In America, size matters. People put a lot of emphasis on body weight, height, and beauty. As a nation, we are conditioned to equate a person's physical characteristics with self-worth. We often associate thin, muscular, and beautiful with strong, self-disciplined, and confident. Conversely, we often look at overweight people as being lazy, ignorant, and weak.

It is not your doing if you think this way, but it is important to recognize how these associations develop. Our families, our friends, and the media impart the message to us at a very early age to judge people by their appearance. As a result, there is an unrealistic perception, not only in this country, but also in other industrialized nations, that if we are thinner, prettier, or more muscular, we can be happier and more successful in our lives.

Q & A

Question: What does the term *negative body image* mean?

Answer: People who have a negative body image have a distorted perception of how they really look. Some women might see their legs as fat or their nose as big when, in reality, they are both average. Those with a negative body image often see other people as more attractive. They somehow equate their "unattractive" appearance to who they really are, causing much anxiety.

BLAME THE MEDIA

Every day we are bombarded with glossy images of sexy models in magazines, on television, and in Hollywood films. Whether it is a supermodel selling lipstick or hawking shaving cream, these images set unrealistic expectations for what we consider "normal" body weight and appearance. For example, from the time they are children, many girls are brainwashed into thinking they should look like the models on TV and in fashion magazines–slim, trim, and a size 0.

For their part, boys are indoctrinated into thinking that all men must have broad shoulders and bulging muscles. An onslaught of advertising images keep coming, chipping away at their self-esteem and body image. Consider some of these studies on the media's effect on body image:

- In a 2006 study, researchers found that 23 animated Walt Disney films associated the attractiveness of 100 female characters with goodness. Think about it for a second: Who is prettier–Snow White or the evil queen? Ariel is thinner and prettier than the evil Ursula.

- In 2000, researchers found that male characters in situation comedies on television were more likely to praise thin female characters than heavier female characters.

- Another study reported that 550 girls from middle-class families were not happy with their body weight and shape. Nearly 70 percent said that the pictures in magazines influenced their perceptions of what a "perfect" body should be. More than 45 percent said those images motivated them to lose weight.

- In a 2002 study of fifth graders, researchers reported that 10-year-old girls were unhappy with their bodies after watching a Britney Spears music video or a segment from the TV show *Friends*.

FRIENDS, FAMILY, AND NEGATIVE TALK

Movies, television, books, and magazines are not the only sources of a person's distorted sense of body image. Parents and friends directly influence perceptions of body image. Whether at home or in school, you are constantly flooded with negative talk about body images. "Look at my thighs; they're so huge." "Yuck, these jeans are too tight on me; I must be getting fat." "I need to go on a diet."

Although you might not think much of it at the time, these comments have a snowballing effect on how you view yourself and other people. In addition to friends and family, health professionals have a responsibility to tell those who are overweight to lose weight. Although their reasons may be valid and they may mean well, the effect can still be devastating.

If you are an athlete, you might feel tremendous pressure to lose weight or **body fat** to perform better or to look more attractive to the judges and the audience. The pressure to lose weight might come from a variety of sources, including coaches, parents, teammates, and yourself. Wrestlers are always trying to "make weight." They will diet until they get down to a particular weight class. This pressure affects and lowers one's self-esteem, sometimes resulting in the development of eating disorders.

AT WHAT COST?

A negative body image can lead to a variety of problems, including depression, low self-esteem, substance abuse, and an unhealthy diet. Having an unhealthy body image also can lead to eating disorders such as anorexia and bulimia. Anorexia is a potentially life-threatening mental illness characterized by severe weight loss caused by self-starvation. In addition to the intense fear of weight gain, anorexia is also marked by a person's distorted image of his or her body.

Those who suffer from bulimia eat massive amounts of food, a process called binging. Once they have binged, bulimics often self-induce vomiting, which is called purging.

Q & A

Question: What does the term *positive body image* mean?

Answer: Those who have a positive body image see their reflection in the mirror as an accurate portrayal of who they really are. That does not mean they do not see their flaws, they simply have a realistic image of how they look. These people are generally more confident than those with a negative body image.

Q & A

Question: I'm a 13-year-old girl, and I don't like the way I look. Will I develop an eating disorder?

Answer: Women and girls who have a negative body image are at greater risk for developing an eating disorder. If a woman develops an eating disorder, she will still have a negative image of her body. Anorexics, for example, often see themselves as grossly overweight, when, in reality, they are very thin.

Q & A

Question: Is it wrong to worry about how I look?

Answer: Caring about one's appearance is perfectly normal. However, it is tough not to cross the line between looking your best and being obsessed with your looks. If a person's preoccupation with looks interferes with normal living, then problems will arise. In such cases, it often helps to see a therapist or health professional for advice about how to restore balance in life.

SELF-HELP TIPS

Studies have shown that enrolling in wellness programs, in which the focus is on healthy bodies (eating healthy foods and exercising) rather than on weight and beauty, can help improve teens' self-image. Eating a proper diet and exercising regularly will make you feel energized. A proper diet not only keeps your body working the way it should, it is also a mental stimulator. In short, exercise makes you feel good about yourself.

According to researchers at the University of California at Los Angeles and other experts, here are some other tips on how to combat a bad body image:

- Love the body you have because you cannot change your basic body type.
- If you have any extra spending money, buy flattering clothes or fitness equipment. Get your hair cut. Do not spend your money on diets.
- Do not weigh yourself. Focus on how well your clothes fit and how good you feel.
- Trying to achieve an unrealistically low body weight might leave you depressed, harming your quality of life.
- Do not compare yourself to others.

■ Exercise will help you feel better. Go for a walk or a swim. Bike or learn how to dance. Take a yoga or aerobics class. Walk the dog or help your parents in the yard.

■ Become friends with people who have a well-balanced attitude about food, weight, and their bodies.

■ Refrain from talking about your weight or the weight of others.

■ Be realistic. Not everyone can look like a swimsuit model or George Clooney. Setting unrealistic goals will impact ways that you can enhance your life.

See also: Anorexia Nervosa; Bulimia Nervosa

FURTHER READING

Davis, Brangien. *What's Real, What's Ideal: Overcoming a Negative Body Image.* Center City, Minn.: Hazelden Publishing & Educational Services, 1999.

McManus, Valerie Rainon. *A Look in the Mirror: Freeing Yourself from the Body Image Blues.* Washington, D.C.: Child and Family Press, 2004.

■ BODY MASS INDEX

A measure of a person's weight in relation to his or her height. The body mass index (BMI) does not measure a person's **body fat** but is a good estimate of a healthy body weight depending on the height of that person. Doctors use BMI to diagnose weight-related problems or potential problems in their patients.

Figuring out if you are overweight, especially if your doctor or another health care professional has said you need to shed a few pounds, is where the body mass index comes in. BMI is a reliable way to find out if you are overweight or even underweight. Although it does not measure your body fat directly, BMI is a good indicator of how much fat your body actually has.

DOING THE MATH

To calculate your BMI in metric units, divide your weight in kilograms by the square of your height in meters. A BMI between 18.5 and 24.9 is considered normal for most people.

Body Mass Index-for-age Percentiles, Boys, 2 to 20 Years

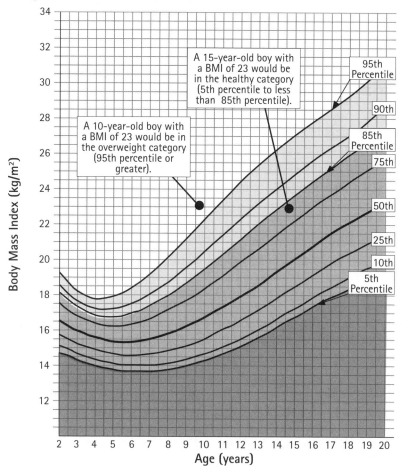

Doctors would classify a 10-year-old boy with a BMI of 23 as obese. They also would classify a 10-year-old with a BMI of 18 as healthy. If your BMI falls on the CDC's chart below the 5th percentile, you are underweight. If your BMI falls between the 5th percentile and less than the 85th percentile, you have a healthy weight. If your BMI falls from the 85th percentile to less than the 95th percentile, you are overweight. If your BMI is equal to or greater than the 95th percentiles, then you are classified as obese.

Source: Centers for Disease Control and Prevention, 2009.

If you want to calculate your BMI using pounds and inches, use this formula: weight (lb) / [height (in)]^2 × 703. In other words, divide your weight in pounds (lbs) by your height in inches (in) squared, and then multiply by a conversion factor of 703. You can also find many BMI charts on the Internet.

Q & A

Question: Is body mass index interpreted differently for children than adults?

Answer: Yes. Although BMI is calculated the same for children and adults, clinicians interpret the data differently. In adults, health officials do not depend on age or gender. For children, those between the ages of two and 20, the BMI growth chart is specific, depending on whether you are a boy or a girl.

Q & A

Question: What is the difference between obese and overweight?

Answer: Obesity is an excessively high amount of body fat in relation to lean body mass. There are various methods to determine the level of fat on a person. In determining whether a person is overweight, a person's body weight needs to be compared to that person's height. An increase in body fat might not be responsible for someone's being overweight. He or she might simply have an increase in lean muscle. For example, a professional athlete who is lean and muscular with very little body fat might weigh more than another person of the same height. Although the athlete is technically "overweight" due to his large mass of muscles, he is not fat.

BODY FAT EXPLAINED

Perhaps you have seen this scenario on television: A person is 30 pounds overweight. To hammer home the point of how much extra fat that person is carrying around, the show's host brings out a white, disgusting, 30-pound cube of animal fat. The person on the receiving end of such news is shocked and mortified at carrying around all that ugly, excess weight.

However, not all fat is bad. Your body needs fat to survive. Fat provides the body with fuel. It insulates and helps the body produce normal **hormone** activity. It assists in transmitting electrical nerve impulses. Too much fat, however, can make you sick and even kill you. People do not want to carry excess fat that burdens the muscles.

The amount of body fat that a person should carry depends on that person. Some people, such as athletes, need less fat to survive. A low percentage of body fat is just enough to provide some athletes with the fuel their bodies need to perform at a high level. Other people, however, need more fat. The Inuit in Alaska, for example, need extra fat because of the extreme cold in the north. The fat acts as an insulating blanket to prevent the loss of body heat in cold climates. Also, a newly pregnant woman needs more fat than a male Olympic swimmer. The extra fat allows the soon-to-be mother to support the growth of the fetus. However, there is a fine line between having enough fat to meet the needs of healthy living and too much fat, which can cause serious health problems.

Researchers have found that people begin to experience health problems when body fat exceeds 22 percent in young men, 25 percent in older men, 32 percent in young women, and 35 percent in older women. Having excess fat is one problem, and where that fat is distributed on the body is another.

Fat that is stored around the organs of the abdomen is more dangerous to a person's health than fat stored elsewhere on the body. When men get older, they tend to store their excess fat in the abdominal region. As women get older, they tend to store fat in the hips and thighs, also known as lower-body fat.

Lower-body fat is relatively harmless. In fact, people who are overweight but tend to store excess fat in places other than the abdomen are less likely to experience health problems than those who store fat near the abdomen.

MEASURING FAT

While BMI gives a good indication of whether you are overweight, other measurements might need to be taken to zero in on specific problems. Health care professionals use several methods to estimate body fat and its distribution. One is *fatfold measures*.

Fatfold measures can provide you with a good estimate of how much body fat you have and where that fat is located. Half of the body's fat lies directly underneath the skin and accurately reflects the total amount of body fat. A skilled health professional uses a specially designed instrument to measure the thickness of the folds of skin on the back of the arm, over the triceps muscle, below the shoulder blade, and in other places. As a person gets fatter, they will see fatfold increase. If the person loses fat, there will be a decrease. Measurements around the abdomen are more reliable than measurements around the upper body.

Another good indicator of fat distribution is the *waist-to-hip ratio*. To calculate the waist-to-hip ratio, divide the waistline measurement by the hip measurement. For example, a woman with a 28-inch waist and 38-inch hips would have a ratio of 0.74. In general, a woman with a waste-to-hip ratio of 0.80 or greater is in the high-risk category for having weight-related health problems, as are men with a waste-to-hip ratio of 0.95 or greater.

Clinicians also use other techniques to determine body composition, including submerging people in water to determine their body density. These are efforts to calculate body fat in order to help people prevent disease.

HEALTH RISKS AND BODY WEIGHT

BMI values go hand in hand with the risks of disease. People with a BMI between 20 and 25 are generally in good health. Those with BMIs that fall below 20 or above 25 are at risk for weight-related diseases. Those below 20 do not have enough fat to sustain a healthy body. Those above 25 have too much fat.

Underweight people can have a variety of health problems. Because they lack the proper nutrients and energy reserves, underweight people will often have a hard time fighting diseases or infections. In fact, most people with cancer die not from the cancer itself, but from **malnutrition**.

For those who are overweight, the health risks are enormous. In fact, obesity itself is classified as a disease. Overweight people often suffer from diabetes, high blood pressure, heart disease, **arthritis**, liver conditions, and a variety of other maladies.

See also: Dieting and Weight Loss; Gender and Nutrition; Nutritional Guidelines and Healthy Diets; Weight Training and Weight Management

FURTHER READING
Centers for Disease Control. "Healthy Weight—It's Not a Diet, It's a Lifestyle." Available online. URL: http://www.cdc.gov/healthy weight/assessing/bmi/childrens_BMI/about_childrens_BMI.html. Accessed on January 27, 2009.

KidsHealth. "Body Mass Index (BMI Charts)." Available online. URL: http://kidshealth.org/parent/food/weight/bmi_charts.html. Accessed on January 27, 2009.

▪ BULIMIA NERVOSA

A mental disorder characterized by periods of overeating, known as binging, followed by self-induced vomiting, known as purging. The American Psychiatric Association classifies bulimics as people who binge or who engage in uncontrolled eating and purging at least twice a week for three months. Bulimics induce vomiting to rid their bodies of all the food they eat. They also abuse **laxatives** and **diuretics**. Some bulimics also exercise excessively.

Because bulimia is a psychological condition, bulimics might feel helpless, anxious, or depressed. They often binge and purge in an attempt to regain some control over their lives. Bulimia is a sign that things have gotten out of control. Bulimics might also be prone to **compulsive** spending and drug or alcohol abuse or find themselves in unhealthy relationships.

Bulimia affects 5 to 10 million girls and women and 1 million boys and men in the United States. Of all bulimics, 90 percent are female. A national survey published in the *American Journal of Psychiatry* in 2001 found that 1.5 percent of women and .5 percent of men said they had been bulimic.

The Youth Risk Behavior Survey, conducted in 2007, asked high school students about the various ways that they tried to lose weight or kept from putting weight on during the 30 days before the survey. Of the teens, 60 percent said they had exercised, and more than 40 percent said they had chosen a diet low on calories and fat. However, some of teens decided to fast, take diet pills, or induce vomiting.

Most bulimics are chronic dieters. They are obsessed with body image. Bulimia, like anorexia, is a major health problem in the United States and in other industrialized countries whose cultures are centered on youth, thinness, success, and control. With counseling, bulimics can get better.

Q & A

Question: Once, my friend and I watched a movie at her house. We stayed up until the early morning hours. We ate a pizza, two bags of

chips, and some cookies. I felt sick afterward. Is this what binging is like?

Answer: No. Binging is much more intense. A true binger lacks self-control. Often, that person is preoccupied with thoughts of food just prior to binging. During the binging episode, that person will usually eat very fast and a lot more food than a pizza, chips, and cookies. A binger might not even feel full after eating substantial amounts of food. Instead of feeling disgusted for eating a lot of food, the binger often feels relieved.

FOOD AS A DRUG

Someone in your class might be a bulimic and you would not know it. Most bulimics stay within five to 10 pounds of their normal weight. They are professional dieters who often gain back the weight after it is lost.

Bulimics use food like a drug. They often feel a "high" by eating vast quantities of food. The food, like an addiction to a drug, numbs and calms the bulimic. Because bulimics are overly concerned about their body and have a strong desire to be thin, they feel as though they must get rid of the food they just ate. They feel as though they need to be punished for such bad behavior. The bulimic will then purge within 30 minutes to an hour after binging. They usually induce vomiting by sticking fingers down their throats. Some use toothbrushes, spoons, or forks.

Purging or excessive exercise is a secret ritual for the bulimic. In fact, a person might be a bulimic for a number of years before telling someone about his or her condition. Mostly, the bulimic knows that something is wrong.

Friends and relatives often suspect something is amiss because they see that large amounts of food are always missing. They also recognize the signs that someone has been purging in the bathroom. When first confronted by family or friends, most bulimics deny they have a problem and become angry and hostile.

A bulimic's dentist might be the first to suspect a patient is suffering from the illness. Vomiting brings up stomach acid. As such, the constant purging damages the teeth. Bulimics often have numerous cavities, and the enamel on their teeth will wear away. They might have a bad throat irritation and chronic hoarseness. Like anorexia, bulimia stresses the body's organs and can damage a person's stomach and kidneys.

WARNING SIGNS ASSOCIATED WITH BULIMIA

Experts say that some of the most common symptoms of bulimia are the following.

- eating uncontrollably
- purging
- strict dieting
- fasting
- vigorous exercise
- vomiting or abusing laxatives or diuretics in an attempt to lose weight
- vomiting blood
- using the bathroom frequently after meals
- preoccupation with body weight
- depression or mood swings
- feeling out of control
- swollen glands in neck and face
- heartburn
- bloating
- indigestion
- constipation
- irregular menstrual cycle
- dental problems
- sore throat
- weakness
- exhaustion
- bloodshot eyes

Fact Or Fiction?

It's important to keep one's weight within the ideal range for one's height, no matter what.

The Facts: While there is no such thing as an ideal weight, there is such a thing as a healthy weight. You can determine your healthy weight by looking at a body mass index (BMI) chart.

Some of the warning signs of bulimia are:

■ a preoccupation with food

■ overeating as a reaction to emotional stress

■ the consumption of huge amounts of food without gaining weight

■ frequent use of the bathroom after meals

■ compulsive exercise

■ swollen cheeks and broken blood vessels in the eyes

Q & A

Question: My sister is three years older than I am and away in college. The last time she came home, she told me about a ritual she and some of her friends have. Every Friday night, they will all meet in a dorm room and buy pizzas, fries, hamburgers, shakes, bags of chips, lots of soda, and boxes of donuts. They sit around talking, laughing, drinking, and eating. After they have eaten all this food, they go into the bathroom and throw up. I'm worried. She says she only does it once a week, and it's not a problem. Should I tell my parents?

Answer: By all means, tell your parents. Your sister is abusing her body. Even though she is now binging and purging once a week, the ritual could evolve into an uncontrollable eating disorder. Go to the library or search the Internet for information on binging and purging. Then give it to your sister. Tell her she is harming her body.

TAKING BULIMIA SERIOUSLY

Doctors take all eating disorders seriously. When a person has symptoms of an eating disorder but does not have specific symptoms of bulimia or anorexia, doctors often diagnose them with the term *eating disorder not otherwise specified*. Although doctors cannot make a specific diagnosis, they understand that something must be done quickly to save the patient's life. The physical and psychological damage people can do to themselves is great. Eventually, the person with symptoms will develop a severe eating disorder.

Those who treat bulimia generally focus on three areas in an attempt to stop the patient from binging and purging:

■ Nutritional rehabilitation. Those who suffer from bulimia will often skip meals and later feel so famished that they binge uncontrollably. Nutritional rehabilitation focuses on setting regular eating patterns. Research shows that those who eat regular meals are less like to experience hunger and therefore feel less deprived. In turn, they are less likely to binge.

■ Psychosocial intervention. Psychosocial intervention is an attempt to work through a bulimic's underlying emotional and psychological problems. Patients often meet with a **psychotherapist**. They also meet in group settings. Psychosocial intervention tries to find ways of improving **self-esteem** and changing attitudes about food, weight, and body image.

■ Medication management. Sometimes **psychotherapy** is not enough to help a bulimic. In some cases, a doctor might prescribe *psychopharmacological drugs,* or drugs that affect the brain and central nervous system. A doctor might also prescribe **antidepressants** to control depression and ease a patient's anxiety and fear. Once the bulimia is under control, medication might also help prevent **relapses.** Relapsing is a major concern among bulimics. Several studies show that after going into **remission,** 25 percent of all bulimics go back to binging and purging in three months. After nine months, however, 49 percent remain in remission.

TEENS SPEAK

Jessica's Story

His name was Michael, and he was the cutest boy in the 10th grade. I was the new kid in school. When I was in middle school, I was as skinny as a "bean pole," or at least that is what my grandmother said. "Eat, eat," she would tell me, shoving a plate of pasta in my face. I ate, so as to not hurt her feelings.

When I graduated middle school, my family and I moved to another town. By that time, I wasn't what you would call skinny, but I certainly wasn't fat. When my clothes got tight, my mom said I was just growing. She would take me out to buy more clothes. My mom was beautiful. She had long blonde hair and a flat stomach. She did the best she could by helping me find clothes that hid my pudgy mid-section. My father would tease me about being a "little pudge ball."

As my sophomore year in high school wore on, I kept on noticing Michael. He played football. He had short, dark hair and a great tan. I was smitten. Finally, after some encouragement by my friends, I walked up to Michael and asked him if he wanted to go out sometime—maybe to the movies. Michael looked at me and said something I have never forgotten. "I don't go out with girls like you," he said. "You're too fat."

I was devastated. I went home and cried and cried and cried. I'd watch TV shows and movies about high school kids. They were always thin and beautiful. They had no trouble getting dates. I fantasized about what it might like to be someone like that. One day my friend Beth and I were watching one of those shows. Beth was skinny. "You know how I keep my weight down?" she said. "I throw up after I eat."

"That's disgusting," I said.

"No, it works," Beth continued. "You should try it. You will get so skinny and hot that Michael will come begging to go out with you."

"You're crazy," I said.

Beth took me to the bathroom and showed me how she made herself vomit. When Beth left that night, I began to think. I do want to be skinny. I do want to lose weight. I want to look like the people on TV. I want Michael to like me. So I began forcing myself to throw up. It wasn't really hard. I felt good afterwards. At first, I ate and vomited once a week. Then I ate and purged twice a week. I was determined to be skinny by the start of my senior year.

See also: Anorexia Nervosa; Body Image; Eating Disorders: Causes, Symptoms, and Diagnoses of; Mental Health and Physical Activity; Obesity

FURTHER READING

Costin, Carolyn. *The Eating Disorder Sourcebook: A Comprehensive Guide to Causes, Treatments and Prevention of Eating Disorders.* 3rd ed. New York: McGraw/Hill, 2007.

Hall, Lindsey, and Leigh Cohn, M.A.T. *Bulimia: A Guide to Recovery.* Carlsbad, Calif.: Gurze Books, 1999.

Normandi, Carol Emery, and Laurelee Roark. *Over It: A Teen's Guide to Getting Beyond Obsessions with Food and Weight:* Novato, Calif.: New World Library, 2001.

■ CALORIES AND WEIGHT

Calories are units of energy in food that, when digested in large amounts, lead to weight gain. Calories come from food. Most Americans eat large portions of food without burning excess calories. That cycle is a recipe for weight gain.

It takes 3,500 excess calories, which get stored in the body as fat, for a person to gain one pound. Therefore, people who consume more calories than the body burns gain weight.

CALORIES ABOUND

You have heard it all before. Do not eat that candy bar; it has too many calories. Do not drink soda that has too many calories. That chocolate cake is loaded with calories. You might even count calories.

What exactly are calories, and how do they get into your body? Most food and drinks contain calories. When you say, "That cookie has 100 calories," you are actually saying that if you ate that cookie, your body would get 100 units of energy.

Calories are not all bad. People need energy to live. What is bad, however, is to ingest more calories than the body needs. When that happens, the body turns excess calories into fat.

The body breaks down **carbohydrates**, fats, and proteins into usable energy. The energy content in food is dependent on how much carbohydrates, fats, and proteins are in the food. Your body gets four calories from every gram of carbohydrates and proteins you eat and nine calories from every gram of fat. That is why excessive fat is unhealthy for you. Most nutritionists recommend that people limit calories from fat to 30 percent or less of their total food intake.

Each person burns calories at a different rate. Still, nutritionists recommend that most children ingest 1,600 to 2,500 calories a day.

Girls in **puberty** need fewer calories than boys. According to the U.S. Food and Drug Administration, girls between the ages of 14 and 18 should consume 1,800 to 2,400 calories a day, depending on how active they are. Boys in that age group should consume 2,200 to 3,200 calories a day. Kids who are more active need more calories than kids who sit and play video games most of the day.

Fact Or Fiction?

Trimming 100 calories a day can make a difference to a person's health.

The Facts: According to the International Food Information Council Foundation (IFIC), cutting 100 calories a day out of your diet could make a difference in how you feel. The IFIC suggests several ways to cut those calories. Share a bag of fries. Replace a tablespoon of regular mayonnaise in tuna salad with a tablespoon of fat-free mayo. To burn off 100 calories, the IFIC recommends walking at a brisk pace for 22 minutes a day. Cleaning the house for 25 minutes also burns calories. Or, to cut calories through a combination of exercise and food, all you have to do is eat five fewer potato chips and walk for six minutes per day.

CALORIES IN

It's easy to find out how many calories there are in the foods you eat. Most food packages have labels that outline the number of calories in that product. Many cookbooks and magazines include nutrition information at the end of every recipe. The burger joint or pizza parlor you go to after school might have a sign with the number of calories for each of the dishes they serve. The library is full of books with nutritional information, as is the Internet.

Knowing about calorie intake can help people make good nutritional decisions. Instead of choosing a piece of cheesecake that contains 300 calories, a person might choose to eat a cupcake with 165 calories. A person who wants to lose weight will be better off eating a banana.

Q & A

Question: I want to lose five pounds. I have tried reducing the number of calories I eat, but it seems not to have worked. What can I do?

Answer: Pay close attention to food portions. The more food you eat, the more calories you will consume, even if the foods are low in fat. Also, exercising regularly is a sure way to lose weight and become a healthier person.

Q & A

Question: What is fiber? Is it important to weight loss?

Answer: You can find fiber in cereals, breads, fruits, and vegetables. Very important in a well-balanced diet, fiber has been found to lower the risks of certain ailments, including heart disease and cancer. The Food and Drug Administration recommends 25 grams of fiber daily based on an intake of 2,000 calories per day.

CALORIES OUT

In addition to counting calories, figuring out how many calories are burned through exercise is a necessity in losing weight. The amount of calories burned depends not only on a person's weight but also on the exercise itself. One of the best ways to burn calories is by swimming or running.

According to the calorie counter at WebMD Health Web site, if you weigh 100 pounds, you can burn 147 calories in 20 minutes by swimming the breaststroke. If you weigh 150 pounds, you can burn 221 calories in 20 minutes. Running burns more calories in that same time period. A 100-pound person running a seven-minute mile burns 207 calories in 20 minutes, and a 150-pound person burns 311.

NATIONAL OBSESSION

Calorie counting, it seems, is a national obsession in the United States. America is fast becoming a nation of overweight people. Bacon cheeseburgers, curly fries, super-sized soft drinks, and two-for-one value meals are making Americans obese. According to the Centers for Disease Control and Prevention (CDC), more than 60 percent of adults in the United States are overweight. The CDC also says that 15 percent of children are overweight. In fact, the CDC blames poor diet and the lack of physical activity for more than 400,000 premature deaths each year in the United States. That is enough people to fill six New Orleans Superdomes.

Overweight people are more likely to develop health problems, such as high blood pressure, heart disease, diabetes, and **arthritis**. Carrying extra weight also means that individuals are more likely to develop various types of cancer, including colon and breast cancers.

Fact Or Fiction?

People who lose weight eventually gain it back.

The Facts: This is fiction. Not everyone who loses weight gains it back, says Rena Wing, a professor of psychiatry at Brown Medical School in Providence, Rhode Island. Wing conducted a research study that shoots holes in this common misconception. The study, known as the National Weight Control Registry, tracked the behavior of 3,000 adults who lost an average of 60 pounds and kept the weight off for an average of six years. Wing concluded that each of these people had four common behaviors that allowed him or her to keep the weight off. These people ate breakfast every day, they were physically active, they frequently monitored their weight, and they ate a low-fat diet.

No one wants to diet. How can eating lettuce and sprouts every day be appetizing? Nutritionists say the best way to lose weight is to enjoy all foods as part of a healthy diet. This includes cutting back on the amount of calories consumed and eating smaller portions—in addition to being physically active. Also, limiting one's intake of beverages high in added sugars helps keep the weight off. There are many calories in sugary drinks and very few nutrients. Nondiet soft drinks, sweetened beverages, and fruit drinks are all examples of foods with a high content of added sugar.

See also: Body Mass Index; Carbohydrates and Exercise; Eating Disorders: Causes, Symptoms, and Diagnoses of; Food Pyramid; Nutritional Guidelines and Healthy Diets

FURTHER READING

Taubes, Gary. *Good Calories, Bad Calories: Fats, Carbs, and the Controversial Science of Diet and Health.* New York: Anchor Books, 2007.

Humphries, Carolyn. *Pocket Calorie Counter.* Berkshire, U.K.: Foulsham Publishing, 2008.

■ CARBOHYDRATES AND EXERCISE

Carbohydrates are any group of **organic** foods that serve as fuel for the body during exercise. Whether running a marathon or step dancing at the gym, foods rich in carbohydrates, such as breads, pastas, fruits, potatoes, and cereals, are what power the body.

Carbohydrates are the food of choice for many professional athletes, including long-distance runners and cyclists. Carbohydrates include sugars, starches, **celluloses,** and **gums.** Carbohydrates are made by **photosynthetic** plants and contain only hydrogen, carbon, and oxygen **compounds.**

CARBS AT WORK

Whether you are quietly sitting at the kitchen table studying for a test or playing a game of basketball, there is a lot going on in your body that allows you either to learn or to run around on the court. While you are studying or setting yourself up for a jump shot, billions of glucose **molecules** in your body are splitting each second to provide you with the energy you need for these activities.

Glucose, which is another word for sugar, and its storage in your body in the form of **glycogen,** provides about half of all the energy the body needs. Every part of the body, from the nervous system to the muscles, needs glucose to function and to remain healthy. The other half of a person's energy comes from fats.

People do not eat glucose or glycogen directly. They come from the foods we eat that are rich in carbohydrates. The body breaks down carbohydrates into energy. The cells use that energy, and excess glucose is stored as fat.

When the body converts carbohydrates into glucose, the pancreas, an organ that sits behind the stomach, releases **insulin,** a **hormone** that allows glucose to enter muscles and other tissues. The body then uses glucose as a source of energy.

Most people who diet try to stay away from carbohydrates. Why? When there is a lot of glucose in the blood, the pancreas produces too much insulin. As such, the body's organs and tissues are inundated with glucose. Eventually, the muscles and tissues can no longer absorb the sugar. The body stores all that extra glucose as fat.

Q & A

Question: How does the body convert carbohydrates into energy?

Answer: First, a person eats foods such as bread and fruit that are loaded with carbohydrates. Next, enzymes break the food down into glucose. The glucose stimulates the pancreas to produce insulin, which allows the glucose to enter muscles and other tissues through receptors. The body's cells then use the glucose for energy. If there is a lot of glucose in a person's system, the body produces too much insulin. This overwhelms the receptors, which lose their ability to absorb glucose into the cells. Because the glucose has to go somewhere, the body stores its excess glucose as fat.

TYPES OF CARBOHYDRATES

Carbohydrates are broken down into two forms: simple and complex. Glucose, fructose, galactose, maltose, sucrose, and lactose are simple sugars. It does not take long for the body to convert these simple sugars into energy. This is why people feel energized rather quickly after eating an orange or drinking an energy drink. Each is a good source of simple carbohydrates.

The body takes a bit longer to digest and absorb complex carbohydrates. Complex carbs provide energy at a much slower rate than simple sugars. Rice, bread, and pasta are foods laden with complex carbohydrates.

Starch is a complex carb and the most important food in the arsenal of an athlete. Starches are stored as glycogen and can be used as fuel during endurance sports.

Q & A

Question: Should I eat before I exercise?

Answer: It is probably not a good idea to eat before exercise. Food in your stomach when exercising might cause an upset stomach, nausea, and cramping. It is best to fully digest a meal before you start exercising. This takes generally one to four hours depending on how much you have eaten. For example, if you are racing in the morning, get up early enough to eat a meal, and eat or drink something that can be digested 20 to 30 minutes before the race. A liquid meal is beneficial just before the start of a race because it is digested easily.

Q & A

Question: What should I eat before exercising or a big race?

Answer: Any type of fresh fruit is good to consume one hour before exercising. Apples, watermelons, grapes, and oranges will provide quick energy. Eat fruit, vegetables, breads, bagels, and low-fat yogurt two to three hours before competition. Fruit, pasta, baked potatoes, energy bars, and sports drinks are good to consume three to four hours before exercising.

THE TRUTH ABOUT BAD CARBS AND GOOD CARBS

Many people used to think that carbohydrates were bad for you. In fact, it was not that long ago that low-carb diets, such as the Atkins Diet and the South Beach Diet, were all the rage. While most nutritionists think that low-carb diets do have their place, it turns out that carbohydrates are not evil. In fact, you could not live without carbohydrates.

Low-carb diets deprive people of fruits and vegetables, which contain phytochemicals, natural substances that help prevent heart disease and cancer. Beta-carotene, which is abundant in orange and yellow fruits, is one of the best-known phytochemicals.

CARB LOADING

Nutritionists say that a healthy diet provides at least 50 percent of our daily energy intake from carbohydrates, 35 percent from fats, and the remainder from proteins. Athletes and those who exercise on a regular basis often "load up" on carbs. In other words, they eat a lot of foods that contain carbohydrates. Runners and cyclists often eat a large plate of pasta the night before a race because pasta is loaded with carbohydrates.

Why do some athletes eat foods rich in carbohydrates? Glycogen is the source of energy that the body uses during exercise. Sprinters and weight lifters use glycogen for intense, short workouts. Glycogen also supplies energy during prolonged exercise, such as jogging. If there is not enough glycogen in a person's system during exercise, he or she will become tired fairly quickly during exercise. If an athlete is fatigued, his or her ability to continue to exercise or compete becomes limited. Therefore, the more carbs he or she eats, the better that competitor will perform.

One study looked at how the body uses glycogen during exercise. The researchers asked people to eat foods low in carbohydrates and high in fat and proteins for three days after intense exercise. Researchers found it took the body's muscles longer to absorb glycogen when eating a low-carb diet. When those in the study were given a diet high in carbohydrates for the same period of time, their muscles were able to absorb much more glycogen at an astounding rate.

The study also found that if people ate a carbohydrate-rich diet for three days prior to exercising while decreasing the intensity of their training, the level of glycogen in the muscles increased dramatically. Health professionals say that the diet of an athlete should contain at least 60 percent carbohydrates.

Another study looked at the influence loading up on carbs had on the performance of long-distance runners. Using a treadmill to simulate a 30-kilometer race, researchers wanted to determine at what point the runners would begin to tire and how manipulation of their diet impacted when they began to feel fatigued.

Scientists divided the runners into two groups after running one 30-kilometer race. The members of one group increased their intake of carbohydrates over seven days, while the other group ate more foods containing fat and protein. Researchers brought the groups back into the laboratory to run another 30-kilometer race.

Scientists found that the group who had loaded up on carbohydrates ran faster during the last 10 kilometers of the simulated race. Eight of the nine runners in the high-carb group documented faster times in the second race compared to the first race.

Carbohydrates are also important to those who play high-intensity sports, such as hockey, tennis, basketball, and soccer. If you have ever played or watched any of these sports, you know that there are quick periods of intense exercise followed by rest or light activity. Although there has been limited research in this area, scientists say the body uses its muscle glycogen rapidly during short periods of high-intensity exercise. Experts say that those who play sports such as soccer can benefit from loading up on foods high in carbohydrates.

Consuming enough carbohydrates helps prevent the body from using protein as energy. If you are not getting enough carbohydrates in your diet, your body will break down protein for glucose. Proteins are generally used by muscles, bone, skin, and hair along with other tissues. If your body is relying on protein for its energy, it impacts your ability to build and maintain muscle, bone, and other tissue. In addition, using protein as energy stresses the kidneys because they have to work harder to eliminate the waste generated by the breakdown of protein.

CARBS AND RECOVERING AFTER EXERCISE

If you run 10 miles, hike up a mountain, or participate in some other strenuous activity, it is very important that you eat more foods with high carbohydrates. When people exercise, tissues and muscles break down and then are repaired. Carbohydrate replacement is important during this recovery process.

The body needs at least four to five grams of carbohydrates after several days to replace glycogen stored in the muscles. However, if you are running or cycling every day, you might need more carbs to help your body repair itself.

See also: Dieting and Weight Loss; Exercise and Strength; Food Pyramid; Nutritional Guidelines and Healthy Diets

FURTHER READING
Wilmore, Jack, David Costill, and Larry W. Kenney. *Physiology of Sport and Exercise.* 4th ed. Champaign, Ill.: Human Kinetics, 2008.
Litt, Ann. *Fuel for Young Athletes: Essential Foods and Fluids for Future Champions.* Champaign, Ill.: Human Kinetics, 2004.

■ DIABETES
See: Blood Sugar, Insulin, and Diabetes; Obesity

■ DIETING AND WEIGHT LOSS
Ingesting food in a regulated manner to help people who are overweight achieve a healthy weight or control their weight. During the past 100 years, the people of the United States have gotten fatter,

while the residents of other nations, such as China, generally remain lean. According to the latest statistics from the Centers for Disease Control, 33 percent of adult American men are obese. That means they have a body mass index (BMI) of greater than or equal to 30. In adult American women, the obesity rate is 35.3 percent. Among children, 16.3 percent are classified as obese.

Why are Americans gaining weight? America is a nation of "couch potatoes," who consume more food energy per individual body weight than they burn. Obesity has many causes, including **genetic,** behavioral, psychological, and metabolic factors. A sedentary, or inactive, lifestyle is partly to blame, as is eating foods that are rich in certain kinds of fat.

In addition to being overeaters, Americans tend also to be dieters. Whether it is the Cabbage Soup Diet, the Grapefruit Diet, or the Hollywood Miracle Diet, Americans are always trying to shed excess pounds. Go online and search under "diet," and you will get 166 million hits.

HOW DO PEOPLE GAIN WEIGHT?

Are you pleased with your body weight? If so, you are in the minority. Many Americans think they should either weigh more or weigh less than they do. However, both being overweight and being underweight have their own health risks.

Calories and fat cells

On its face, gaining weight is a simple process. People consume much more energy, namely calories, than they burn. Calories are units of energy in food that, when digested in large amounts, lead to weight gain. To gain a pound, you have to eat an extra 3,500 calories without burning those calories off through exercise.

When we consume more calories than we burn, we store that excess energy in the fat cells of our bodies. The amount of fat on a person's body correlates to the number and size of the fat cells. Those fat cells can grow, and continue to grow. When they reach their maximum size, the cells divide, creating more fat cells. When someone loses weight, the size of that person's fat cells decreases, although the number of fat cells stays the same. That is why many people with extra fat cells tend to regain weight rapidly after having shed extra pounds. When they regain the weight, their shrunken fat cells expand.

Genes

A person's **genes** also play a role in weight gain. Genes are inherited characteristics, such as eye and hair color. If both parents are obese, there is an 80 percent chance that their children also will be obese. When neither parent is obese, there is less than a 10 percent chance that their children will be fat. Genetics also influences the way we burn our energy. Researchers have recently located a gene in humans named the *obese gene*. The gene regulates the amount of fat in the body.

Overeating

In addition to overeating, inactivity is another reason why our waist-lines are expanding. Obese people who are inactive will gain weight even though they might eat *less* than thinner people.

The inactivity associated with watching television or sitting in front of a computer for hours at a time is another major factor why some people gain weight. One study reports that watching television lowers the amount of energy we expend and cuts into the time we have to be active. You cannot play sports or ride a bike if you are sitting in the living room watching cartoons or *American Idol*. Watching television also increases the amount of snacks we eat. Children who watch too much television are most at risk. Obesity increases by 2 percent for each additional hour of TV viewing.

DIET FADS AND SOCIAL PRESSURE

You have seen the commercials or read the advertisements: "Lose Weight Now!" "I lost 20 pounds in six weeks; so can you!" Sports stars, movie stars, and everyday people hawk the latest weight-loss fads. It could be a pill. It might be a treadmill. It could be a weight-loss program or diet fad that promises quick, easy weight loss. No matter what the product or the gimmick, Americans spend between $30 to $40 billion to shed weight each year.

Some 30 to 40 percent of all women in the United States and 20 to 25 percent of all men are trying to lose weight at any given time. However, the sad truth is that only 5 percent of all people who try to lose weight keep the weight off. The pressure is enormous, because our culture places a high value on thinness.

Overweight people often face discrimination and prejudice in many aspects of life. Thin people often consider overweight people

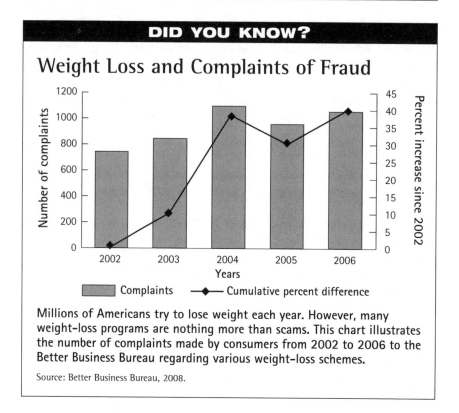

DID YOU KNOW?

Weight Loss and Complaints of Fraud

Millions of Americans try to lose weight each year. However, many weight-loss programs are nothing more than scams. This chart illustrates the number of complaints made by consumers from 2002 to 2006 to the Better Business Bureau regarding various weight-loss schemes.

Source: Better Business Bureau, 2008.

lazy and lacking in self-control. Overweight people pay more for health insurance and clothing. Many find it difficult to find comfortable seating in airplanes; they sometimes have to purchase two tickets instead of one. Colleges are less likely to admit overweight people, and employers are less likely to hire people with weight problems. Researchers say if you are an overweight woman, the cultural and social problems associated with obesity are magnified. Overweight people tend to die younger for a variety of reasons and have severe health problems throughout their lives, including high blood pressure, diabetes, heart problems, **stroke,** and liver and gallbladder diseases.

There are many factors to consider when deciding whether a person needs to lose weight, including consulting a doctor or other health care professional. Those factors include the extent of someone's obesity, age, health, and genetic makeup. Not all overweight people are unhealthy, just as not all thin people are healthy.

DIETS, DIETS, EVERYWHERE

The Rice Diet, the Scarsdale Diet, the Zone Diet . . . diets are everywhere. What do weight loss diets do? For one thing, diets restrict the intake of specific foods. The Atkins Diet, for example, recommends that people eat more protein while avoiding carbohydrates. However, what works for one person—if it works at all—might not work for anyone else. Moreover, many dieters look for a quick solution to their weight problems. They want their pounds to melt away while they are asleep. Although no one has invented a pill that will allow you to "burn" the weight away, some dieters do take pills and supplements.

DIETING DANGERS

In the weight loss world, there is one true maxim: "Dieters beware." Many diets exaggerate claims. Fad diets, for example, often lie about weight loss. In fact, following some fad diets is more hazardous than being overweight. Those on a fad diet might end up with health problems as simple as headaches or as serious as death.

Fad diets abound. How would you enjoy eating hamburgers and steak for breakfast, with a side order of beef jerky? Sounds like a meat lover's heaven, right? In fact, it is part of a diet that limits carbohydrates.

Low-carb diets were the rage several years ago, when, among others, talk show host Oprah Winfrey featured a book titled *The Carbohydrate Addictions Lifespan Program* on her show. The book outlined a weight loss program high in proteins and low in carbohydrates. Proteins are nutrients found in meat, fish, dairy products, grains, nuts, and legumes. They are important in maintaining and repairing tissue. Carbohydrates are nutrients found in fruits, grains, and vegetables.

Those who follow low-carb diets say that millions of people are carbohydrate addicts. In other words, they cannot stop eating foods high in carbohydrates, just as a drug addict cannot stop getting high. When they eat foods rich in carbs, the body of the carbohydrate addict produces too much insulin. Insulin is the hormone that allows **glucose** to enter the muscles. The muscles become overwhelmed with insulin and are no longer able to absorb all of the glucose. As a result, the body stores the excess glucose as fat. By reducing the amount of carbohydrates in a person's diet, supporters of the low-carb diets argue, the body reduces the amount of insulin and therefore the amount of fat in the body.

Critics have said that low-carb diets are unhealthy. They say that the extra insulin is triggered not by excess carbs, but by being too heavy in the first place. Low-carb diets also deprive people of fruits and vegetables, which have beneficial nutrients.

According to the Food and Drug Administration (FDA), you should ask questions before you start a weight loss program. The FDA recommends asking these questions.

- What are the health risks associated with this diet?
- What data are there that prove the diet or program actually works?
- Do people keep off the weight after they leave the diet program?
- Are there any costs for membership, weekly fees, food, supplements, maintenance, and counseling? What is the payment schedule? Does health insurance cover any of these costs? Can I get a refund if I drop out of the program?
- Does the diet program have a maintenance program? Does that program cost extra?
- What kind of professional supervision does the company provide? What are the credentials of these professionals?
- What are the program's requirements? Are there special menus or foods, counseling visits, or exercise plans?

The FDA says that if a diet is too good to be true, then it probably is. The agency recommends keeping clear of diets that promise "easy," "effortless," "guaranteed," or "miraculous" results. Dieters beware.

Q & A

Question: How much weight do I need to lose to be in good health?

Answer: Losing small amounts of weight in a healthy way is very beneficial. Losing 5 percent of your body weight can improve your blood pressure and cholesterol levels. They key is to make small changes in your eating and exercise habits.

WEIGHT CYCLING

Many dieters fall into a trap called *weight cycling,* or endless rounds of weight loss and weight gain. Weight cycling is also known as "yo-yo" dieting because the weight keeps going up and down, just like the toy. When people repeatedly lose weight and gain it back again, their bodies become very good at making and storing fat. Each attempt to lose weight becomes harder and longer. Gaining weight, however, gets easier.

The psychology of weight cycling goes like this: "I am overweight and unhappy. I would like to be happy. If I lose weight, I will be happy. My goal is unrealistic, and I try too hard. I lose a little weight but then gain it back. I am overweight and unhappy." Some research shows that it might be healthier to maintain a slightly overweight body than go through these constant weight fluctuations.

Q & A

Question: I see diet pill ads on TV all the time. Are they worth the money?

Answer: Generally not. Diet pills do not lead to permanent weight loss. The best method for losing weight is to follow good eating and exercise habits.

THE RIGHT WAY TO DIET

The best way to diet is to seek advice from a professional, such as a licensed dietitian or nutritionist. He or she will set up a specific diet tailored to your needs. A good dietician will take your health history and come up with a diet that is well suited for any medical problems you might have. He or she will also coordinate your diet with your lifestyle.

In theory, while you are on a diet, you should not lose more than one pound a week, although everyone's body is different. Experts recommend counting calories and eating a balanced diet. Eat foods that are naturally high in fiber, such as fruits and vegetables.

Limit the intake of high-fat foods, such as butter, cheese, and whole milk. Avoid sweets, for example, and have a salad. Remember that regular exercise is as important as nutrition when trying to lose or maintain weight.

See also: Body Image; Body Mass Index; Calories and Weight; Eating Disorders: Causes, Symptoms, and Diagnoses of; Food Groups; Food Pyramid; Obesity; Sports Drinks and Energy Bars

FURTHER READING

Gay, Kathlyn. *The Scoop on What to Eat: What You Should Know About Diet and Nutrition* (Issues in Focus Today). Berkeley Heights, N.J.: Enslow Publishers, 2009.

Shanley, Ellen, and Colleen Thompson. *Fueling the Teen Machine.* Palo Alto, Calif.: Bull Publishing, 2001.

■ DISEASE AND FITNESS

The relationship between illness and lack of exercise. Extensive research has shown that physical activity, even at the most moderate levels, promotes good health and prevents disease. Researchers say that 75 percent of adults in the United States are sporadically active or completely inactive. The lack of physical activity can result in many diseases, including high blood pressure, heat disease, obesity, lung disease, and diabetes.

In children, inactivity has reached epidemic proportions. The Centers for Disease Control and Prevention (CDC) reports that the number of obese children aged six to 11 has risen from 6.5 percent between the years 1976 and 1980 to 17 percent between 2003 and 2006. The CDC also says that the percentage of children who participate in daily school or extracurricular physical education classes has dropped from 42 percent in 1991 to 28 percent in 2003.

You do not have to be an athlete to reap the benefits of physical activity, neither do you have to run marathons or hike up mountains. Experts agree that any physical activity can be beneficial. Researchers say that people should exercise 20 to 60 minutes per day three to five days per week. Pulling weeds in the garden, walking the dog, or even climbing the stairs at school all add to the recommended time a person should spend being active each day.

WHAT IS FITNESS?

At its most basic level, experts define *fitness* as "the characteristics that enable the body to perform physical activity," according to the book *Understanding Nutrition.* What are these characteristics? They include the flexibility of joints and the strength of the body's muscles, including the heart.

In a much broader sense, physical fitness means meeting physical demands and having reserve energy left over. Still another definition of physical fitness relates to the body's ability to withstand stress.

For people to be physically fit, they must exercise enough to develop the flexibility, strength, and endurance to meet the challenges of life and to achieve a reasonable body weight. Furthermore, there has to be energy left over. Flexibility allows the joints to move freely without risk of injury. Strength and endurance help the muscles work longer and fatigue less. Exercise builds up lung capacity and strengthens the heart muscles.

AEROBIC AND ANAEROBIC EXERCISE

There are many ways to exercise. You can jog, bike, or swim. You can play soccer, shoot baskets, or just walk around the block. Most physical activity falls into two categories, **aerobic** and **anaerobic**.

Aerobic means "with oxygen" and refers to how the body uses oxygen in the **metabolic,** or energy-generating, process. Aerobic exercises involve improving the body's ability to consume oxygen. During aerobic exercise, the body breaks down **glycogen** to form **glucose.** Glycogen stores short-term energy and releases that energy when the body needs it the most. The body stores glycogen in the liver and muscles.

When performed correctly, aerobic exercise maximizes the body's ability to use oxygen. It also makes the body's **cardiovascular** and respiratory systems stronger and more efficient. Aerobic exercise also tones and shapes the body. Aerobic activities include, among other things, tennis, aerobic dancing, jumping rope, and swimming. Aerobic exercises are done at a moderate, continuous pace over a long period.

Anaerobic exercise deals with power, agility, and strength. Working out with weights is a type of anaerobic activity. The duration of anaerobic exercise is usually short and depends on the body's ability to break down glucose without oxygen. Anaerobic activity makes the muscles stronger and body more flexible but does very little for the heart and lungs.

Fact Or Fiction?

You will burn more calories if you exercise longer and at a lower intensity.

The Facts: The faster you walk, jog, or bike, the more calories you burn. The key is to start slow and gradually increase your activity. Research shows that low to moderate workout routines are good for you.

TEENS AND PHYSICAL ACTIVITY

It was not long ago that many teenagers were lean and physically fit. Before the industrial age, most people lived on farms. Young people would work hard in the morning and then work hard again in the afternoon when they came home from school—if they went to school at all. Most of the food they ate came directly from the farm. There were no such things as high-calorie processed food. No Devil Dogs or Twinkies. Fast food restaurants did not exist. There were no televisions to watch or video games to play.

With industrialization and modern conveniences, life got increasingly easier for children. Today, most teenagers and children live a very sedentary, or physically inactive, lifestyle. When was the last time you walked to school? Most students take a bus or ride in a car. Children rarely ride from place to place on bicycles. Instead, someone drives them to where they need to go. There is always more television to watch and more computer games to play. Children rarely play outside. As a result, they have become less physically active. As they become less active, they are becoming increasingly overweight, and in greater numbers. Many children are obese. According to a 2000 study by the CDC, lack of physical activity has contributed to a 100 percent increase in child obesity in the United States since 1980.

Consider these facts from the American Heart Association.

- Overweight adolescents and children are more likely to suffer from high blood pressure, high **cholesterol**, and type 2 diabetes.
- Overweight children and adolescents are more likely to become obese adults.
- There is a direct link between obesity and poor school performance.
- There is a link between obesity and substance abuse, premature sexual behavior, and physical inactivity.
- Obese children are more at risk later on in life for chronic diseases such as **stroke**, cancer, muscle and bone disorders, and gallbladder disease.

Q & A

Question: I don't like to play sports. How can I be physically active?

Answer: You can exercise without joining a team. A brisk walk for about 20 minutes a day is a good way to keep fit. Ride a bike, or help your parents in the garden or around the yard. Even walking around the mall is a good way to exercise. Swimming, in-line skating, cheerleading, skateboarding, practicing martial arts, and horseback riding are some of the best ways to keep trim and fit. Also, playing Frisbee in a park with your friends is a form of exercise.

Q & A

Question: I'm skinny. Do I need to exercise?

Answer: You certainly do. Being thin does not mean you are healthy. While obesity is associated with disease, being thin alone will not keep you safe from possibly suffering a heart attack, stroke, or a number of serious illnesses.

Q & A

Question: Can I exercise too much?

Answer: Yes. If you are just starting to exercise, you should rest every other day, or, at the very least, alternate your physical training: Work your arm muscles one day and run the next. You are probably exercising too much if you become easily fatigued, have a decrease in performance, or have muscle soreness and damage.

WHY EXERCISE?

Your body responds to a lack of physical activity in many ways. Your body becomes weak. As such, it becomes harder to fight diseases and infections. You also lose muscle mass. There is hope, however. All you have to do is put down the video game controller and get off the couch. If you are still not convinced that exercise is good for you, here are some benefits of regular physical activity.

■ The ability to enjoy a restful sleep. After exercise, sleeps occurs naturally. During rest, your body repairs itself and gets rid of the wastes generated by exercise. The body also rebuilds itself during rest, making you a stronger person.

■ Better nutritional health. When you exercise, your body burns energy. By eating wisely, active people consume more nutrients. They are less likely to have problems associated with a bad diet and inactivity.

■ Limiting your **body fat.** Exercise helps maintain a lean body while helping you slim down. Active people have less body fat than inactive people.

■ Fighting diseases and infections. Fitness strengthens your body's immune system, which allows it to better battle diseases and viruses.

■ Better lung and heart functions. Your heart and lungs will become stronger. As such, your body will better utilize oxygen.

■ Limiting your risks of diabetes. Exercise regulates your body's blood sugar and the creation of insulin.

■ Having a long life. Exercise will increase your chances of having a long, high-quality life. Active people have a lower death rate than inactive people. A fast-paced walk around the block each day can add years to your life.

EXERCISE AND MENTAL HEALTH

Exercise will not only help get your body in shape, it also will improve your mind. Studies show that if you are feeling depressed, shooting hoops or swimming laps will help chase away the blues.

For example, a few years ago, a Canadian psychologist concluded that a physical fitness program is just as effective in treating clinical depression as **psychotherapy.** People with clinical depression are usually sad and have feelings of worthlessness. Some clinically depressed people also harbor thoughts of suicide. Greg Tkachuk, a professor of psychology at the University of Manitoba, found that aerobic and anaerobic exercise could relieve depression. He suspects that physical activity spurs the production of **serotonin,** a brain chemical that affects a person's mood.

Researchers say that it might take at least 30 minutes of exercise a day, three to five days a week, to improve a person's symptoms of depression. Exercise also helps boosts a person's confidence, provide healthy coping skills, and give a person a chance to meet or socialize with others who are also exercising.

Fact Or Fiction?

I don't have to watch what I eat if I'm constantly exercising.

The Fact: Eating a proper diet is just as important as exercise in maintaining a healthy body.

HOW TO GET STARTED

Now that you know that exercise can help you avoid many diseases, the next step is getting started. Here are some ideas.

- Pick an activity that you like to do. Chances are, you will continue to do it.

- Try not to start out too fast. Gradually work your way up to 30 minutes a day by adding a few minutes each day to your activity.

- The more you exercise, the easier it gets. Periodically increase the length, time, or intensity of the activity. For example, the first time you walk around the block, it might take you 40 minutes. The next time, try to complete the circuit in 35 minutes, and then 30 minutes after that. If you are jogging around a track, start off walking, then gradually increase the distance and speed.

- Join a team or a group. It is usually fun to exercise with other people. People encourage each other and often have helpful hints. If you do not want to join a team, it can be fun to play basketball, tennis, or other games with your friends.

- Keep track of your activities, and set goals. You will see improvements in your body and health in just a few short weeks. It is very rewarding to achieve a goal when you are exercising.

Keep in mind that every little bit helps. Perhaps you can walk to school a few times a week. If you take a city bus to get around town, get off a few blocks from your destination, then walk the rest of the way. Take the dog for a walk every night. Play outside with your friends. Get up and move around. It takes very little to begin reaping the health benefits of physical activity.

Fact Or Fiction?

I lift weights. If I stop, my muscles will turn to fat.

The Facts: Muscle and fat are not the same. You cannot turn fat into muscle, and you cannot turn muscle into fat. If you stop working out, your muscle tissue will shrink. You might feel flabbier, but you are not fatter. When your muscles get smaller, they do not need as many calories. As such, your **metabolism** slows. When your metabolism slows, you might gain body fat if you eat the same amount of calories.

See also: Aerobic Exercise, Types and Benefits of; Blood Sugar, Insulin, and Diabetes; Body Mass Index; Mental Health and Physical Activity

FURTHER READING

Shryer, Donna. *Body Fuel: A Guide to Good Nutrition* (Food and Fitness). Tarrytown, N.Y.: Marshall Cavendish, 2007.

Favor, Lesli J. *Weighing In: Nutrition and Weight Management* (Food and Fitness). Tarrytown, N.Y.: Marshall Cavendish, 2007.

■ EATING DISORDERS: CAUSES, SYMPTOMS, AND DIAGNOSES OF

Psychological disorders characterized by an obsession with food, weight, and eating. Health professionals consider eating disorders, such as anorexia nervosa and bulimia nervosa, diseases because they have predictable symptoms and outcomes.

Many factors are involved when looking for causes of an eating disorder. Mental health, peer pressure, family issues, **genetics**, society, and the media all can play a role. More than 8 million Americans suffer from some type of eating disorder. Almost half of all Americans know someone who has an eating disorder. Eating disorders affect people of all races and backgrounds. While many consider eating disorders a female problem, millions of men also suffer from the disease. Doctors and health care professionals can treat eating disorders. Psychologists, nutritionists, and others have treated millions successfully.

People who suffer from eating disorders often try to hide their illnesses. They spend an inordinate amount of time thinking about what to eat and how to keep their affliction secret. Those suffering from anorexia often wear baggy clothes or even put weights in their pockets before they weigh themselves at a doctor's office. People who binge are likely to eat normally in public. Once they are alone, however, they will find ways to eat huge quantities of food. Those who purge by inducing vomiting will often look for out-of-the-way bathrooms so no one can hear what they are doing. Nevertheless, the physical signs of an eating disorder will become apparent over time.

WHO GETS SICK?

Although eating disorders can happen any time in life, most cases occur during childhood and adolescence. In 1997, the Centers for Disease Control and Prevention (CDC) reported that 4.5 percent of high school students induced vomiting after meals or used **laxatives** to control their weight. Experts say the actual number is much higher because many eating disorder cases are underreported. For example, those suffering from bulimia are able to hide their purging and often do not become noticeably underweight.

Anorexia is the third most common **chronic** illness in adolescent women, after **asthma** and obesity. Researchers estimate than anorexia occurs in 0.5 to 3 percent of all teenagers.

While eating disorders affect both men and women, women seem to suffer the most. Some studies report that 90 percent of eating disorder patients are women. In addition, the number of men reporting an eating disorder is on the rise. In 2000, a Minnesota health survey reported that 13 percent of teenage girls and 7 percent of teenage boys have an eating disorder. While most eating disorder studies focus on middle-class Caucasian females, new studies are reporting that eating disorders are increasingly affecting Hispanics and African Americans.

COMMON EATING DISORDERS

Anorexia and bulimia are two of the more common eating disorders. Anorexia is a chronic, potentially life-threatening mental illness characterized by severe weight loss caused by self-starvation. Anorexics have an intense fear of weight gain and a distorted body image. They often deny that they are hungry.

People who suffer from anorexia often ignore hunger signals, thereby controlling their desire to eat, yet they may be preoccupied with food. They might cook for themselves or others. There are two types of anorexia. One type is called *restricting anorexia.* Restricting anorexia is the classic form of the condition. People with this subtype maintain their low body weights by carefully regulating the food they eat and by excessively exercising and starving themselves.

Binging and purging is a subtype of anorexia, whereby individuals restrict their food intake by binge eating. Once they have binged, these individuals often self-induce vomiting, or purging. Others also misuse laxatives, **diuretics,** or enemas to rid themselves of food and avoid any weight gain. The difference between this form of anorexia and bulimia is that bulimics are classified as those who binge and purge at least twice a week for three months, according to the American Psychiatric Association.

Anorexia is most common in females and usually begins in adolescence. Between 1 and 2 percent of all females develop anorexia.

Bulimics may feel helpless, anxious, or depressed. They often binge and purge in an attempt to regain some control over their lives. Those who suffer from bulimia may also be prone to **compulsive** spending, drug or alcohol abuse, or find themselves in unhealthy relationships. Most bulimics are chronic dieters who are obsessed about their body image.

CAUSES

Why do people have eating disorders? The reasons vary. Some suffer from depression, loneliness, and low **self-esteem.** Others may abuse drugs and alcohol or have deep-seated feelings of inadequacy.

In December 2004, the American Psychiatric Association published a study that examined how often anxiety disorders occur in anorexics and bulimics. Anxiety disorders are mental conditions characterized by excessive fear and dread. Anxiety disorders recur from time to time. They are also long lasting. Researchers found that about two-thirds of the patients they studied had an anxiety disorder, such as a panic disorder or a phobia, as well as an eating disorder. Most developed anxiety disorders when they were children, years before their eating disorders took hold.

In 2008, researchers at the University of Virginia reported that girls with attention deficit/hyperactivity disorder (ADHD) might have a "substantially greater risk" of developing symptoms of bulimia. Girls with ADHD are impulsive, which might make it harder for them to maintain healthy eating habits, researchers said.

Individuals who are often complimented on the way they look or made fun of because of their weight or sexual development are also at greater risk of having an eating disorder. Victims of sexual or physical abuse are also likely to develop eating disorder symptoms. Eventually, the eating disorder begins to define the patient's identity, making it very difficult for the individual to let go of the disorder.

FAMILY INFLUENCES

Often, unhealthy family relationships trigger eating disorders. Children whose parents were not nurturing or supportive often develop an eating disorder. Those children will have self-esteem issues. Still, even children who had a loving, nurturing family can suffer from an eating disorder. Parents may overemphasize thinness or exercise without realizing the destructive nature of their actions at the time. These parents usually have extremely high expectations of their children.

Also, overprotective parents may harm their children by smothering them. An overprotected child often turns to eating and exercising as a way to assert independence and gain some control over his or her life.

Girls with separation anxiety often fall prey to eating disorders. Some girls become anorexic because they do not want to separate from their parents, even to go to school. Children who have mothers who also suffer from eating disorders are more likely to develop eating disorders themselves. According to researchers, a mother who has an eating disorder has an unhealthy view about nutrition and food consumption and often passes down those negative views to her children. Sibling rivalry or the desire to be like a brother or sister might also play a role in the advance of the disorder.

GENETIC CAUSES

A person's **genes** may also be a factor in developing an eating disorder. Genes are the tiny pieces of biological material parents pass down to their children. Genes determine inherited characteristics such as eye and hair color. In 2006, scientists at the University of North Carolina at Chapel Hill studied 30,000 Swedish twins. They concluded that there were genetic links in 56 percent of anorexia cases they studied.

In 2007 in another twin study, researchers concluded that genes played a role in eating disorders in girls between the ages of 14 and 18. Five years earlier, researchers reported that anyone whose mother or sister suffers from an eating disorder is 12 times more likely to become an anorexic and four times more likely to become a bulimic.

Fact Or Fiction?

Anyone with an eating disorder has an addiction.

The Facts: That is not entirely the case. Not all people with eating disorders have an addictive personality, in which people habitually give in to a physical or psychological need for something, such as drugs or tobacco. However, for some, an addictive personality can contribute to an eating disorder.

Fact Or Fiction?

Certain personality traits, such as being a perfectionist or being obsessive or compulsive, cause eating disorders.

The Facts: This is a fact. Perfectionists usually set extremely high standards for themselves and others. Although you might look at someone as a high achiever, that person might regard his or her accomplishments as inadequate.

MEDIA INFLUENCES

The influence of the media in industrialized nations, such as the United States, also plays a role in the development of eating disorders. Every day the media bombards teenagers with images of thin women and men who seemingly have the perfect body types. Whether teens are looking at the advertisements in magazines, watching television, or viewing a movie, society is hammering home the point that thin is better.

As such, many teens will do anything to achieve the perfect body. Although the average American woman weighs 140 pounds and stands 5' 4" tall, the average female model weighs a paltry 117 pounds and is 5' 11" tall. The media's influence on society has been a subject of intense study for decades.

Researchers from a study at Harvard Medical School looked at the small Pacific island population of Fiji before and after the arrival of television. Before TV came to the island in 1995, most of those living on Fiji thought that the ideal body was round, slightly flabby, and soft. The islanders watched American television shows for three years. After that, the residents of Fiji changed their attitudes. Teenage girls came down with symptoms of eating disorders. The study also found that female islanders who watched TV three or more nights a week were 50 percent more likely to feel "too fat" than those who watched less TV.

The media distort a person's body image. Fat is bad, and thin is good. Fat is ugly, and thin is sexy. Thin people are successful and happy, fat people are not. In 2000, researchers found that male characters in situation comedies on television were more likely to praise thin female characters than heavier female characters. Another study reported that 550 girls from middle-class families were not happy with their body weights and shapes. Nearly 70 percent said that pictures in magazines influenced their concepts of what a "perfect" body should be like. More than 45 percent said those images motivated them to lose weight.

Q & A

Question: Will I get an eating disorder because I am a teenager?

Answer: While an eating disorder can strike anyone at any time, many teens are in danger. A study by the National Women's Health Resource Center reported that 90 percent of those diagnosed with bulimia or anorexia usually develop the affliction between the ages of 12 and 25. Teenage girls are more susceptible than teenage boys.

SYMPTOMS

You think a friend of yours might have an eating disorder, but you cannot be sure. Experts say that some of the most common symptoms of bulimia are:

- uncontrollable eating
- purging
- strict dieting
- fasting
- vigorous exercise

■ vomiting or abusing laxatives or diuretics in an attempt to lose weight

■ vomiting blood

■ using the bathroom frequently after meals

If someone you know has a preoccupation with body weight; is depressed or has wide mood swings; and is always complaining about heartburn, indigestion, or constipation, he or she might be suffering from bulimia. Girls suffering from an irregular menstrual cycle also might be bulimic.

Anorexics can have many health problems, including hair loss, bruising, lack of sleep, and fatigue. Moreover, anorexics often abuse drugs and alcohol. Some studies suggest that between 12 percent and 18 percent of those who suffer from anorexia have substance abuse problems. Anorexia also decreases a woman's chance of having a baby. A pregnant woman with anorexia faces a high risk of having a miscarriage, a **Cesarean section,** or an infant with a low birth weight or birth defects.

Ultimately, eating disorders can result in death. The suicide rate for anorexics totals half of all anorexic deaths in the United States. Many bulimics and anorexics die from complications resulting from **malnutrition.**

See also: Anorexia Nervosa; Body Image; Bulimia Nervosa

FURTHER READING

Nelson, Tammy. *What's Eating You?: A Workbook for Teens with Anorexia, Bulimia & Other Eating Disorders.* Oakland, Calif.: New Harbinger Publications, 2008.

Orr, Tamra, B. *When the Mirror Lies: Anorexia, Bulimia, and Other Eating Disorders,* New York: Franklin Watts, 2007.

Herzog, David B., and Debra L. Franko. *Unlocking the Mysteries of Eating Disorders* (Harvard Medical School Guides). New York: McGraw Hill, 2007.

■ EXERCISE AND INJURIES

Injuries caused by participating in sports or other forms of exercise. Most such injuries are caused by repetitive motion; they occur when a certain part of the body is overused.

Many runners often suffer injuries, such as pulled leg muscles, while other athletes suffer from tennis elbow. Doctors use the term *sports injury* to describe injuries obtained during sports or exercise. Some injuries occur because of poor training practices or lack of physical conditioning. Other injuries occur because of improper equipment. You can also injure yourself by not warming up properly before an activity.

Although you can hurt any part of your body while exercising or playing sports, sports injuries usually affect impact a person's muscles, bones, joints, and tissues, such as **cartilage**. Some athletes also suffer brain and spinal cord injuries.

There are two types of exercise- or sports-related injuries. *Traumatic* injuries, such as head injuries, muscle strains, and fractures, often occur in contact sports, such as football and rugby. *Overuse* injuries, such as shin splints in runners, develop over time.

HOW COMMON ARE SPORTS INJURIES?

Whether you are playing an organized sport, such as lacrosse or field hockey, or playing basketball in the backyard, injuries are common for those who exercise. Injuries can occur during any activity, such as biking, swimming, weight lifting, and jogging. Injuries also can occur during recreational activities, such as boating.

Every day in the United States, emergency room doctors treat more than 10,000 people for injuries sustained through exercise or activity, according to the Centers for Disease Control and Prevention (CDC). Emergency room doctors treat an estimated 1.5 million people a year for injuries sustained while exercising or playing a sport. More than 715,000 exercise- or sports-related injuries occur each year in schools. Children get hurt the most, accounting for an estimated 40 percent of all emergency room visits. Because adolescents and young adults (under the age of 25) participate in sports- and exercise-related activities the most, they account for a third of all sports-related injuries, according to the CDC.

CAN SOMEONE BE TOO ACTIVE?

According to some doctors, the answer is "yes." In recent years, doctors have seen an upswing in sports-related injuries in children because, in their opinion, parents are pushing their kids to train too hard. In 1975, Lyle Micheli and several other doctors at Children's Hospital in Boston set up the first U.S. clinic devoted to kids who were hurt playing sports. Back then, Micheli told *Sports Illustrated* that most of his

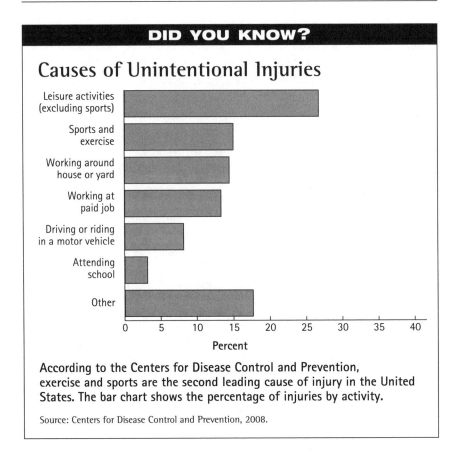

DID YOU KNOW?

Causes of Unintentional Injuries

According to the Centers for Disease Control and Prevention, exercise and sports are the second leading cause of injury in the United States. The bar chart shows the percentage of injuries by activity.

Source: Centers for Disease Control and Prevention, 2008.

patients suffered common injuries, such as sprains and muscle pulls. Today, however, overtraining is causing most of the injuries Micheli and his colleagues treat. Micheli estimates that 75 percent of the children he sees at his clinic hurt themselves by training and playing too hard and too fast. Overuse injuries often occur in sports such as baseball, basketball, running, gymnastics, and swimming. Shoulder and arm overuse injuries involve throwing, while running and jumping injuries often strain the legs or feet. Golfers, tennis players, and gymnasts often suffer hand and wrists injuries through overuse.

One type of overuse injury centers on a child's "growth plate." The growth plate is located at the ends of long bones in the arms and legs, areas of growing tissue. That tissue is ultrasensitive. When a child trains too much, he or she stresses the growth plate, which often results in stress fractures, broken bones of the lower legs and feet.

Children who are not used to physical activity and then start exercising regularly are also prone to overuse injuries. However, athletes can prevent most overuse injuries by making sure they schedule periods of rest into their sports routine. Micheli says the responsibility for these injuries rests not with the children but with parents who push their kids too long and too hard.

The American Academy of Pediatrics has issued guidelines to reduce overuse sports injuries.

- Choose an age-appropriate sport. The academy says children should be at least six years old before playing team sports.

- Get into shape before beginning a sport. This includes having a doctor examine you before you start exercising. Also, it is a good idea to talk to your doctor about what kind of conditioning program you should be on. Conditioning might include stretching, endurance training, and **aerobic** exercise.

- Properly warm up before playing baseball, running, or participating in any activity. Stretching and other warm-up exercises can reduce injuries. Cooling down at the end of a game is also important.

- Don't overdo it. When you are participating in an activity for the first time, start out slowly and gradually increase as you go on. If you grow tired or start to feel pain, take some time off to recover.

- Keep hydrated by drinking a lot of water or sports drinks. **Dehydration** causes fatigue and increases the chance of injury.

- Wear good athletic shoes. No matter what sport or exercise activity you are participating in, good athletic shoes that fit well will cut down on the number of injuries you might sustain.

- See a doctor right away if you are injured.

COMMON SPORTS INJURIES

These are some of the most common sports injuries, according to the National Institutes of Health.

■ Sprains and strains. A sprain occurs when an athlete stretches or tears a **ligament,** the strong connective tissue, made up of the protein **collagen,** that joins bones together. Ligaments prevent you from dislocating your bones but allow you to flex your joints. Sprains occur during a fall or blow to the body that knocks a joint out of position. Ligaments can also tear. Ankles, wrists, and knees are prone to sprains. Strains occur when you twist, pull, or tear a muscle or **tendon.** Tendons connect muscle to bone.

■ Knee injuries. Knee injuries are very common in sports. Each year, more than 5.5 million people see a doctor because they have hurt their knees. The knee is a complex joint. Sometimes the injury can be minor; other times it is more severe. One of the most severe knee injuries is a torn *anterior cruciate ligament,* or ACL. The ACL keeps the knee stabilized during movement and connects the thigh bone to the tibia, the larger of the two lower leg bones. Like a thick rubber band, the ACL prevents the thigh bone, or femur, from sliding over the top of the tibia during sudden stops and quick pivots, the moves generally associated with basketball players and football running backs and wide receivers. A blow to the knee or an improper fall can damage the knee.

■ Fractures. Broken legs, arms, fingers, and toes can occur anytime during sports or exercise. A fracture is a break in a bone due to a quick, one-time injury, such as being tackled on the football field. Bones can also break because of repeated stress, called stress fractures. Some fractures are clean, while others might be compound fractures, which occur when the bone punctures the skin.

■ Dislocations. Dislocations occur when two bones that are joined become separated. Dislocations occur frequently in contact sports such as football.

■ Shin splints. Shin splints are common among runners. The term refers to pain along the tibia, or shinbone.

■ Achilles tendon injuries. A torn Achilles heel is one of the most painful injuries an athlete can have. The

Achilles tendon connects the calf muscle to the back of the heel. The injuries are so sudden and painful that professional football players have been known to shout out in pain when they injure one.

HEAD INJURIES

It's Monday night football. The linebackers blitz from the right side and up the middle. The offensive line does all it can to stop the rush of the oncoming giants. Although the guards do their best, they cannot keep the quarterback protected much longer.

The quarterback scrambles but is blindsided by a charging opponent, who tackles the quarterback with vengeance. The quarterback goes down; his head strikes the hard field. He does not get up. He is knocked out for a brief time. When his teammates place him on a stretcher, the gridiron giant does not know where he is. He just received a **concussion.**

A concussion is a mild traumatic brain injury. Concussions are common in sports, especially contact sports such as football, although skiers, gymnasts, and horseback riders also often sustain concussions during falls. Of college football players, 10 percent receive concussions each season, while 20 percent of high school players sustain brain injuries each season.

TEENS SPEAK

My Last Football Game

My name is Andy, and I love to play sports. I'm not one of those jocks you see in the hallway. I'm a backyard athlete. In other words, I have a little talent, but not enough to play organized sports where everyone is much better. I play basketball, baseball, street hockey just for fun with my friends. We keep active, and we have a good time.

I used to play touch football. One day last fall, my friends and I went to the local park for a game of touch football. We were playing five on five. We generally play football when the NFL is in season. Afterwards, we get pizza and watch the games.

The field was wet and muddy this particular Sunday morning, just the way we like it. We were playing for about a half hour. My team was leading. Then the play happened. I was lined up as a receiver on the left side of the offensive line. My friend Dave was on the other team. His job was to guard me to make sure I didn't catch the ball. The play we had set up was fairly simple. I was to sprint straight for 10 yards, then right toward the middle of the field. Jack, the quarterback, promised to hit me directly in the chest with the football.

Jack lined up behind the center. The center hiked the ball. Jack took the ball and dropped back to pass. Once the ball was hiked, I sprinted directly toward Dave. I faked him with my shoulders and gained a step and half. I motored toward the middle of the field. As I sprinted, I looked toward Jack, the quarterback. He saw how open I was. All I had to do was catch the ball and turn up field for the touchdown. Jack's pass was right on the mark. It hit me square in the chest. I tried to cradle the ball with my hands, but it slipped from my grasp. The ball fell with a thud to the muddy field. I had dropped the pass.

I was so mad with myself that I tried to kick the ball as it bounced up from the field after I dropped it. I missed. I slipped on the mud and came down hard on my left ankle. I fell to the ground in pain. After a few moments, I tried to stand up with the help of my friends. I could not put any weight on the ankle. I was in so much pain.

I went to the doctor the next day. My ankle was very swollen and black and blue. He X-rayed the ankle. There was no break. He said I had sprained my ankle. There was really nothing he could do. He gave me an air splint and told me to put ice on it several times a day. After about three days, the swelling started to go down. I wished I had broken the ankle. That way the doctor could have set the fracture. The sprain was awfully painful for a very long time.

Today, when I'm walking or hiking with my dogs, my ankle will suddenly twist on itself, and I'll trip or tumble to the ground. It hasn't been the same since. By the way, that was the last time I played football.

TREATING INJURIES

Some sports injuries are **acute**. They happen suddenly and can be severe. A sprained ankle is an example of an acute injury. Some of the symptoms of an acute injury include sudden, intense pain, swelling, or a break in a bone.

Other injuries are **chronic**. They happen over time and through overusing one area of the body. The pain associated with chronic injuries occurs when performing an activity or as a dull ache when you are resting.

There are times when you will need to see a doctor when you are injured. Many times, you can treat certain types of sports injuries at home. It is wise to seek medical treatment when the injury causes severe pain, swelling, or numbness. Also, seek treatment if you cannot put weight on the impacted area. Sometimes you will need to seek treatment or see a doctor for an old, nagging injury that flares up from time to time.

You can treat your injuries at home if they are minor. Rest is the key to treating some injuries. Reducing your activity gives the affected area a chance to heal. You should apply ice to an injured area for only 20 minutes at a time, four to eight times a day. Keeping an injured ankle, knee, or elbow elevated helps decrease swelling. Sometimes, though, you might have to seek medical treatment when home treatments do not work. Many injuries can be prevented, or the damage lessened if it occurs, by wearing protective gear such as helmets and using authorized equipment.

See also: Aerobic Exercise, Types and Benefits of; Exercise and Strength; Weight Training and Weight Management

FURTHER READING

Bellenire, Karen, ed. *Sports Injuries Information for Teens.* Detroit: Omnigraphics, 2008.

Spilling, Michael, ed. *Sports Injuries: How to Prevent, Diagnose & Treat.* Broomall, Pa.: Mason Crest Publishers, 2004.

■ EXERCISE AND STRENGTH

The relationship between anaerobic exercise, or strength training, and muscle power and agility. The most common definition for strength is "the ability to exert a force against a resistance." Certain types of athletes, such as sprinters and weight lifters, need strength training to be at the top of their game. Bench pressing weights, tossing the javelin, and running the 100-meter dash are types of anaerobic activities. Such high-intensity, short-duration exercises depend on the body's ability to break down **glucose** without oxygen.

Exercises that increase a person's strength should not be confused with **aerobic** activities, such as tennis, aerobic dancing, jumping rope, and swimming. Unlike anaerobic exercises, aerobic activities are done at a moderate, continuous pace over a long period. Aerobic exercises are designed to make the body use oxygen more efficiently and strengthen your lungs and heart.

Strength exercises work the body's muscles against extra weight, known as resistance. Resistance training increases the amount of muscle mass in the body by making the muscles work harder. In addition to building muscle, strength exercises also help burn calories, decreasing body weight.

Q & A

Question: My older brother, who works out at the gym, often tells me that his technique is important. What does he mean?

Answer: The way someone lifts weights is called technique. When lifting weights or doing any other strength-related exercises, you must do the exercise correctly. Failure to keep your hands, legs, and body in the correct positions could lead to an injury.

WELL-ROUNDED WORKOUT

Gaining strength is not easy. In order to build muscle strength, people generally have to work out with weights. There are two different types of weights people use. Some people use *free weights,* which include barbells, dumbbells, and hand weights. Others use *weight machines.* While free weights work specific groups of muscles individually, weight machines let you work on one specific muscle at a time.

Still, strength exercises are not dependent on weights. You can use your own body weight as resistance by doing push-ups, sit-ups, and squats. You can also do **isometric** exercises to build strength. During isometric exercise, the muscles contract against an immovable force.

People tend to use a combination of free weights, weight machines, and their own bodies when working out. Experts say athletes should incorporate their strength training into a well-balanced workout routine that also includes aerobic exercises.

THE SCIENCE OF STRENGTH

How exactly does strength training work? Every muscle in the body has one job—to contract. Whether it is curling a 50-pound dumbbell or waving good-bye to a friend, your body's muscles use their power to contract, or they do not contract at all. Unlike the heart muscles and lung muscles, which contract involuntarily, the body's skeletal muscles can contract only by the force of a person's will. For example, every time you raise your hand in class, you are making a voluntary, or conscious, decision to move your arm muscles.

When you exercise using the various methods of strength training, your body's muscles work hard against whatever form of resistance you happen to be using. The cells of the body react to the extra resistance by becoming bigger and stronger. That allows your muscles to contract more efficiently.

There are many benefits related to strength training. Obviously, you will become stronger. As you get stronger, you will be able to do much more strenuous activities. Strength training reduces **body fat,** and resistance training also increases the density of bone while building muscle.

By using and increasing muscle mass, a person also can increase the energy that the body uses at rest and during activity. The more muscle you have, the more energy your body burns to function properly. As such, your body burns more calories and fat. As you burn more fat, your body becomes leaner. Resistance training also improves the heart and circulatory system.

Strength exercises also help the elderly improve their health as they battle such conditions as **arthritis.** Researchers at Tufts University in Massachusetts completed a study of older men and women with moderate to severe osteoarthritis in their knees. The subjects of the study completed a 16-week strength training program. Researchers reported that 43 percent of those studied had an increase in muscle strength and a general decrease in the disabling effects of the disease. Researchers concluded that working out eased the pain of the arthritis more than medication.

Weight training can also help people with type 2 diabetes. Studies show that those who completed a 16-week strength training program improved their bodies's ability to control glucose, or blood sugar. Not only did the subjects of the study become stronger, they gained muscle, lost body fat, and were more self-confidant.

Strength training, like other exercise, helps control depression. It also improves the ability of people to get a good night's rest.

Q & A

Question: I have a medical condition. Can I still do strength training?

Answer: There is probably some type of strength exercise that you can do that will not impact your health. You should talk to your doctor and discuss your specific conditions and goals. Your doctor can make the necessary recommendations.

METHODS OF STRENGTH EXERCISES

Weight training uses stacks of weights to oppose the contraction of the muscles. There are different weight training exercises designed for specific muscle groups. When you use weights, the majority of the resistance comes when your muscles contract in order to lift the weight. The muscles must overcome the inertia, or resistance, of the heavy objects. Performing constant repetitions allows the muscles to continually battle against the resistance of the weight.

The idea of resistance training is to gradually overload the muscles so they get stronger. Using exercise machines, swimming machines, and types of isometric exercises builds up the body's muscles.

HOW TO GET STARTED

If you are interested in a strength training routine, you should consult a doctor to make sure that your body can handle the stress. Once your doctor gives you the go-ahead to exercise, consult an expert, such as a personal trainer or coach, to tailor a workout that is specific to your needs. He or she will tell you how to work out, when to work out, and what kinds of warm-up and cool-down activities you should do.

Once you have a workout plan, begin slowly so your body can adjust to the activity. Chances are that you will wake up the next morning good and sore. Do not be alarmed. That is very natural.

If you are working out with free weights or weight machines in a gym or at home, make sure that someone is there to "spot" you, known as a spotter. He or she not only acts as a coach who encour-

DID YOU KNOW?

Recommended Exercises

Type of Physical Activity	Age Group	
	Children	Adolescents
Moderate-intensity aerobic	■ Active recreation such as hiking, skateboarding, rollerblading ■ Bicycle riding ■ Walking to school	■ Active recreation, such as canoeing, hiking, cross-country skiing, skateboarding, and rollerblading ■ Brisk walking ■ Bicycle riding (stationary or road bike) ■ House and yard work, such as sweeping or pushing a lawn mower ■ Playing games that require catching and throwing, such as baseball, softball, basketball, and volleyball
Vigorous-intensity aerobic	■ Active games involving running and chasing, such as tag ■ Bicycle riding ■ Jumping rope ■ Martial arts, such as karate ■ Running	■ Active games involving running and chasing, such as flag football, and soccer ■ Bicycle riding ■ Jumping rope ■ Martial arts, such as karate ■ Running

(continues)

DID YOU KNOW? (CONTINUED)

- Sports such as ice or field hockey, basketball, swimming, tennis, and gymnastics

- Sports such as tennis, ice or field hockey, basketball, and swimming
- Vigorous dancing
- Aerobics
- Cheerleading or gymnastics

Muscle-strengthening

- Games such as tug of war
- Modified push-ups (with knees on the floor)
- Resistance exercises using body weight or resistance bands
- Rope or tree climbing
- Sit-ups
- Swinging on playground equipment/bars
- Gymnastics

- Games such as tug of war
- Push-ups
- Resistance exercises with exercise bands, weight machines, and hand-held weights
- Rock climbing
- Sit-ups
- Cheerleading or gymnastics

Bone-strengthening

- Games such as hop-scotch
- Hopping, skipping, and jumping
- Jumping rope
- Running
- Sports such as gymnastics, basketball, volleyball, and tennis

- Hopping, skipping, jumping
- Jumping rope
- Running
- Sports such as gymnastics, basketball, volleyball and tennis

These are some of the physical activities recommended by the Centers for Disease Control and Prevention to help children and adolescents become healthier. Included in the list are both aerobic and anaerobic exercises.

Source: Centers for Disease Control and Prevention, 2008.

ages you but also will be able to tell you if you are not doing a particular exercise correctly. Having a spotter with you is also safer than working out alone. Accidents can happen even in the gym.

Q & A

Question: Can I make my own weights for working out?

Answer: It is not advisable to make your own weights. Plastic jugs filled with sand or a five-pound bag of sugar are not designed for weight training. They can easily break and injure you.

Most fitness experts say if you are just starting out in the gym, you should train three days a week for 20 minutes to one hour. They also recommend that you work one muscle group per day: arms one day, legs the next, your chest the day after.

Limber muscles will help you work out. Stretch or ride a stationary bike for 20 minutes before you begin working out. Being flexible will help you avoid injury.

Be careful when working out. Take your time and have fun. You can track your progress and see how much stronger you become with each workout. Still, there are a few things to watch out for. You are still growing. As such, your bones, joints, and **tendons** are still developing. It is easy to strain or pull muscles and **ligaments**. If you are in the middle of an exercise and something feels out of place—stop! Pain is your body's way of telling you that something is wrong. Get checked out by a doctor before you resume your routine.

While weight training is important, it should not be a person's only form of exercise. Your heart and lungs need to work out, too. As stated before, combine anaerobic exercises with aerobic exercises.

See also: Aerobic Exercise, Types and Benefits; Exercise and Injuries; Weight Training and Weight Management

FURTHER READING

Gaede, Katrina, Alan Lachica, and Doug Werner. *Fitness Training for Girls: A Teen Girl's Guide to Resistance Training, Cardiovascular Conditioning, and Nutrition.* Chula Vista, Calif.: Tracks Publishing, 2001.

Rioppetoe, Mark, and Lon Kilgore. *Starting Strength*. 2nd ed. Wichita Falls, Tex.: The Aasgaard Company, 2007.

■ FATS

A group of **organic compounds** (made up of carbon, hydrogen, and oxygen) that are a source of energy in foods. Fats belong to a group of substances called **lipids**. One of six nutrients found in the diet, they are either solid or liquid. Like the nutrients proteins and carbohydrates, fats also supply calories to the body. In fact, fat provides more than twice the number of calories than do proteins and carbohydrates.

At first glance, the word *fat* might sound bad. However, if the body is to work properly, it needs some fat each day. Fat provides essential fatty acids, which the body does not manufacture. Fatty acids can be found only in food and are important for controlling inflammation and blood clots.

Fat also serves as the storage bin for the body's extra calories. Fat helps insulate the body against the cold and is an important source of energy. When the body has used up all its calories from carbohydrates, which generally happens during the first 20 minutes of exercise, the body begins to drain calories from fat. Without fat, you would not have healthy skin or hair. Fat also helps the body absorb certain vitamins, including vitamins A, D, E, and K.

Some foods have plenty of fat, including nuts, oils, butter, and meat. Other foods, such as fruits and vegetables, have no fat whatsoever. While advertisements on television and in magazines tout products as "low fat" or "fat free," nutrition experts warn that some fat is not only good for your health, it also helps people satisfy their appetite so they do not eat as much food.

Health experts have always preached that eating less fat is a good way to lose weight and control certain diseases. While a fat-free diet has helped many individuals, the low-fat approach really has not helped America become a leaner, less obese nation.

According to the Harvard School of Public Health, in the 1960s, Americans ate enough fat to supply them with about 45 percent of their daily calories. At the time, only 13 percent of Americans were considered obese, and less than 1 percent of the population had type 2 diabetes.

Fast forward to 2009. Today, although Americans have reduced their fat intake to 33 percent of their daily calories, 34 percent of

Americans are obese, and 8 percent suffer from type 2 diabetes. Harvard researchers say that cutting fat from the diet does little to curb weight or stop disease. What really matters, researchers say, is the type of fats people eat.

TWO MAJOR FATS

There are "good" fats and "bad" fats. Good fats are beneficial for the heart and the body's other organs. Bad fats not only cause weight gain but contribute to many health problems.

Unsaturated fats are good fats. You can find unsaturated fats in some oils and fish. The best unsaturated fat is found in olive oil, peanut oil, canola oil, albacore tuna, and salmon.

Saturated fats are bad fats. Our bodies make all the unsaturated fat we need. We do not need any additional saturated fat. Meat and other animal products, such as milk (except for skim), butter, and cheese, contain saturated fats. If you eat too much saturated fat, you can raise your blood's **cholesterol** levels, which increases the risk of heart disease. Health experts say it is a good idea to limit the intake of saturated fats.

THE BATTLE OVER TRANS FAT

Trans fat is a "really bad" bad fat. Trans fats can raise blood cholesterol levels and increase the risk of heart disease. Trans fats are found in potato chips, and snack foods, and baked goods, including donuts and cupcakes. Most fried food is laden with trans fats. On average, people eat about six grams of trans fats a day. However, most people should eat less than two grams a day and zero grams if possible.

Many communities, including New York City, have banned restaurants from cooking with trans fat oils. Eliminating trans fats has been a big topic of study and debate in recent years. A Harvard School of Public Health study linked trans fats to heart disease. Since New York City banned trans fats, other communities, such as Philadelphia, also have enacted bans.

According to Harvard's Walter Willett, the Fredrick John Stare Professor of Epidemiology and Nutrition and chair of the school's Department of Nutrition, regulations banning trans fat oils will significantly reduce the rates of heart attacks, **strokes**, type 2 diabetes, and other health problems. "We estimate that if we replaced all the trans fats in the American diet with polyunsaturated fats from vegetable sources, we could reduce the national risk of type 2 diabetes by up to 40 percent," Willett reports.

Why not ban butter and dairy products, too? Willet says these foods have too little trans fat in them. In fact, most of the calories in these foods come from saturated fat. Although they may not be good for your heart and should be eaten in moderation, they are not as bad as trans fat.

TRIGLYCERIDES

Most of the body's fat consists of *triglycerides,* the chief form of fat in a person's diet. Triglycerides provide the body with energy. When a long-distance runner is racing in a marathon, the athlete's stored triglycerides provide the fuel that keeps him or her moving. When you lose your appetite for whatever reason, triglycerides fuel your body until you can eat again.

Without stored fat in the form of triglycerides, people could not survive. Because fat is not a good conductor of heat, the stored fat under the skin keeps people warm in cold climates. Layers of fat inside the body cushion the organs against sudden shocks and jolts.

Fat also helps the body use its two other sources of energy, carbohydrates and proteins, more efficiently. The body releases energy when fat combines with **glucose.** That process spares the body from raiding the stores of energy in protein. A lack of protein can have dire consequences for one's health.

Fact Or Fiction?

Fat-free and low-fat foods can solve the obesity problem in the United States.

The Facts: While these foods can help manage the amount of fat and calories we eat, maintaining weight has to do more with using as many calories as we consume. To achieve a healthy weight, a person must eat fewer calories and burn calories through exercise.

HOW MUCH FAT IS OKAY?

For years, the world's health experts at the American Heart Association, the National Institutes of Health, and the World Health Organization called on people to limit their fat intake to 30 percent of their daily calories. Problems arose when people stopped eating fat altogether—even the good fats.

Recent studies have shown that low-fat diets do not prevent heart disease. A study published on February 8, 2006, in the *Journal of the American Medical Association* found that 49,000 women had the same rates of heart attack, stroke, and other forms of **cardiovascular** disease regardless of whether they followed a low-fat diet.

The eight-year study, called the Women's Health Initiative Dietary Modification Trial, divided the women into two groups. One group ate a low-fat diet, and the other group continued to eat what they normally ate. The study concluded that women on the low-fat diet did not lose— or gain—any more weight than those who were not on a low-fat diet.

Still, experts say that children who are two years or older should get 30 percent of their daily calories from fat. The Federal Food and Drug Administration also recommends that adults get 30 percent of their calories each day from fat.

See also: Calories and Weight; Carbohydrates and Exercise; Food Groups; Food Pyramid

FURTHER READING

Enig, Mary, G. *Know Your Fats: The Complete Primer for Understanding the Nutrition of Fats, Oils and Cholesterol*. Bethesda, Md.: Bethesda Press, 2000.

Erasmus, Udo. *Fats That Heal, Fats That Kill*. Burnaby, British Columbia: Alive Books, 1993.

Sears, Barry. *When Good Fat Turns Bad*. Nashville: Thomas Nelson, Inc. 2008.

■ FOOD GROUPS

In a diet, a family of foods that share similar nutritional properties. Until recently, there were four basic food groups. However, as science and American lives have changed, so have the groupings of food we eat. Now there are six food groups. They include grains, fruits, vegetables, dairy, meat and protein, and fats and oils, including sweets.

Grains are probably the most important food group. Grains include a variety of food, such as cereal, rice, pasta, whole wheat bread, and rolls. Every day you should eat at least six to 11 servings from this group. Grains provide much-needed carbohydrates, which our bodies use for fuel.

DID YOU KNOW?

Recommended Dietary Allowance for Protein

	Grams of protein needed each day
Children ages 1–3	13
Children ages 4–8	19
Children ages 9–13	34
Girls ages 14–18	46
Boys ages 14–18	52
Women ages 19–70+	46
Men ages 19–70+	56

Source: Centers for Disease Control and Prevention, 2008.

Fruits include apples, apricots, bananas, strawberries, and many others. Vegetables include carrots, broccoli, green beans, potatoes, and spinach, and many others. Fruits and vegetables provide fiber in our diets as well as vitamins and minerals. Fiber helps the body digest food. You should eat three to five servings of fruits and vegetables each day.

Dairy includes milk, cheese, and yogurt. Dairy is a good source of calcium, which our bones need to remain strong. It is important to have two to four servings each day.

Meats include poultry, fish, and beef. Meat is a good source of protein, iron, and zinc. Our bodies use protein as a source of energy and as its main building blocks, providing the nutrients for strong muscles, bone, healthy hair, and **cartilage.**

The least important food group includes fats, oils, and sweets. The foods in this group provide little nutritional value and should be eaten sparingly.

DIETARY GUIDELINES

Eating a balanced diet—consuming small portions from each of the food groups—is essential for good health. The United States Department of Agriculture (USDA) began issuing dietary guidelines in 1894. The USDA updates these guidelines every five years. According to the guidelines issued in 2005, to achieve the highest nutritional impact, the USDA encourage people to:

- Eat two cups of fruit and two and a half cups of vegetables per day. These amounts could fluctuate depending on calorie level.

- Eat a total of six ounces of grains a day, with half coming from whole-grain products.

- Eat a variety of fruits and vegetables each day. The USDA recommends eating different colors of fruits and vegetables several times a week.

- Consume three cups per day of fat-free or low-fat milk or equivalent milk products.

- Consume less than 10 percent of your daily caloric intake from **saturated fat,** while keeping your total fat intake to 20 to 35 percent. Most fats should come from unsaturated fats found in fish, nuts, and vegetable oils.

- Limit your intake of salt and sugar, along with fats and oils high in saturated and/or trans fatty acids.

You can find the full list of these guidelines at http://www.healthierus.gov/dietaryguidelines.

Q & A

Question: What is the difference between "good" carbs and "bad" carbs?

Answer: Many diet books talk about good carbs and bad carbs. The term *good carbs* refers to foods that have more fiber and complex carbohydrates, which take more time to break down into glucose. *Bad carbs* are carbohydrates in food made from white flour and added sugars. The USDA recommends eating fiber-rich carbohydrates found in the vegetable, fruit, and grain groups. Avoid added sugars.

The key to maintaining a balanced diet is simply to eat a lot of fruits, vegetables, whole grains, and low-fat or fat-free dairy products. You can supplement your diet with lean meats, poultry, fish, eggs, and nuts. Eat foods that are low in saturated fats, trans fats, **cholesterol,** sodium (salt), and added sugars.

See also: Calories and Weight; Carbohydrates and Exercise; Dieting and Weight Loss; Fats; Food Pyramid; Nutritional Guidelines and Healthy Diets

FURTHER READING

Bellenir, Karen. *Diet Information for Teens: Health Tips About Diet and Nutrition, Including Facts About Dietary Guidelines, Food Groups, Nutrients, Healthy Meals, Snacks and Weight Control* (Teen Health Series). Detroit: Omnigraphics, 2006.

Schlosser, Eric, and Charles Wilson. *Chew on This: Everything You Don't Want to Know About Fast Food.* New York: Houghton Mifflin, 2006.

■ FOOD PYRAMID

A graphic depiction of the six main food groups. The U.S. government designed the Food Pyramid in an attempt to make it easier to understand how to eat healthy. Consumers will often see various representations of the Food Pyramid on boxes or containers of food.

The U.S. Department of Agriculture (USDA) first designed the Food Pyramid in the 1960s, when it consisted of only four food groups. Each food group was stacked on top of another, with the most important food groups located at the wide end of the pyramid. As the years progressed, however, the USDA added more groups. In 2005, the USDA replaced its old Food Pyramid with a new graphic designed to do a better of job of informing Americans about what constitutes a healthy diet.

Called MyPyramid, the new Food Pyramid is less specific than previous Food Pyramids. To read more specifics, log on to http://mypyramid. gov. This highly interactive site is packed with nutritional information and advice. The site also will provide you with recommendations on eating a well-balanced diet specifically tailored to your needs. The site takes into account your age, weight, height, and activity level.

CLIMBING THE PYRAMID

Nutritional experts designed the MyPyramid illustration to depict the ideal variety, moderation, and daily proportions of the six major food groups. The amount a person needs is indicated by the width of the bands. The stairs represent physical activity.

The new food pyramid, called MyPyramid, symbolizes a personalized approach to healthy eating and physical activity. The wider base stands for foods with little or no solid fats or added sugars; these

MyPyramid, 2005

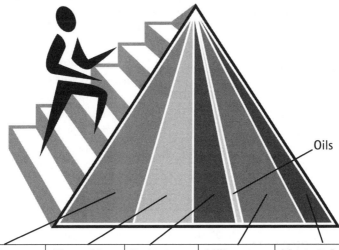

Oils

Grains	Vegetables	Fruits	Milk	Meats & Beans
Eat at least 3 oz. of whole-grain cereals, rice, or pasta every day.	Eat more dark-green veggies like broccoli, spinach, and other dark, leafy greens.	Eat a variety of fruits.	Go low-fat or fat-free when you choose milk, yogurt, and other milk products.	Choose low-fat or lean meats and poultry.
	Eat more orange vege-tables like car-rots and sweet potatoes.	Choose fresh, frozen, canned, or dried fruit.	If you don't or can't consume milk, choose lactose-free products or other calcium sources.	Bake it, broil it, or grill it.
	Eat more dry beans and peas like pinto beans, kidney beans, and lentils.	Go easy on fruit juices.		Vary your pro-tein routine— choose more fish, beans, peas, nuts, and seeds.

For a 2,000-calorie diet, you need the amounts below from each food group.

• Eat 6 oz. every day.	• Eat 2 ½ cups every day.	• Eat 2 cups every day.	• Get 3 cups every day; for kids aged 2 to 8, it's 2.	• Eat 5 ½ oz. every day.

The new food pyramid, called MyPyramid, symbolizes a personalized approach to healthy eating and physical activity. The wider base stands for foods with little or no solid fats or added sugars; these should be selected more often. The narrower top stands for foods with more added sugars or fats. The more active a person is, the more of these foods can be consumed. In other words, find your balance between food and physical activity.

Source: U. S. Department of Agriculture, April, 2005.

should be selected more often. The narrower top stands for foods with more added sugars or fats. The more active a person is, the more of these foods can be consumed. In other words, find your balance between food and physical activity.

The bands in the pyramid start out wide at the bottom and narrow toward the top. This represents *moderation.* The wider base stands for foods in the group that have little or no solid fats or added sugars. You should select these foods more often than foods that contain some fats or added sugars. For example, it is less healthy to eat a piece of cherry pie at the top of the fruit group because of the added sugar and fat. The cherry itself would be at the bottom of the fruit group because cherries are part of a healthy diet.

The width of each band represents, in a generalized way, how much food from that group a person should eat each day as part of a balanced diet. The width of the oil food group is very thin. In other words, you should limit your intake of this food group.

See also: Calories and Weight; Carbohydrates and Exercise; Dieting and Weight Loss; Nutritional Guidelines and Healthy Diets

FURTHER READING

D'Elgin, Tershia. *What Should I Eat? A Complete Guide to the New Food Pyramid.* New York: Ballantine Books, 2005.
Ward, Elizabeth. *The Pocket Idiot's Guide to the New Food Pyramid.* New York: Alpha Books, 2005.

■ GENDER AND NUTRITION

Dietary habits based on the differences between males and females. Men and women are very different when it comes to certain aspects of life. While men and women have many things in common, the nutritional needs of each gender vary, especially when it comes to teenage boys and girls. Men seem to be able to eat more than women without gaining weight, and men lose weight more easily than women. Therefore, the recommended daily dietary intake for men and women, and boys and girls, tends to differ.

Every day people make decisions about what types of foods to eat. Each decision cannot really help or hurt in the short term. However, if a person makes the same decisions every day for decades, the rewards or the problems associated with those decisions are likely to impact one's life. There are a variety of reasons why we make certain food choices. We choose foods based on our individual tastes, traditions, and social and cultural influences as well as on perceived nutritional content. First, we eat certain foods because they taste good, especially those that are sweet or salty. We also eat foods out of habit. Many people have toast for breakfast simply because they have been doing so for years.

Cultural traditions also play a role in what types of food people eat. Every country in the world has its own eating traditions. In addition, the United States is a culinary melting pot, with seemingly innumerable choices for food. Indian food, Thai food, Mexican food, and Chinese food abound. There is no shortage of food in the United States.

Moreover, each region of the country has its own traditions. In New England, lobster and other seafood are favorites. In the South, grits, hushpuppies, and collard greens are always on the menu.

Convenience and economy, emotional comfort, and religious and social values also affect the types of food we choose. For example, when people are running late to school or work, they often choose fast food because it is convenient and cheap. Many religions have rules on what types of foods to consume. Moreover, some people might avoid certain foods because of the way they are prepared for sale.

Finally, people eat certain foods because of their nutritional benefits. While pizza tastes wonderful on a Friday night, some people still prefer a salad.

TEENS AND NUTRITION

As teenagers, your nutritional requirements are much different than the requirements of your parents or grandparents. Nutritional requirements also vary depending on gender.

Adolescent bodies are constantly changing, transforming themselves from biological children to biological adults. These changes are happening all the time. Children between the ages of eight and 13 gain an average of 6.5 pounds (2.96 kilograms) each year. They also grow two inches per year.

Each person matures differently on a physical level. During **puberty,** the body starts making **hormones.** Those hormones spark physical changes, such as muscle growth and changes in height and weight, and male and female bodies have different proportions of muscle and fat. Most teens will gain weight rapidly during this period. As long as **body fat,** muscle, and bone are in the right proportion to one another, the body grows normally. As adolescents grow, the systems that run the body, including the central nervous system, also mature. The growing body needs the right fuel to support this rapid physical development, which means that teenagers need additional calories, protein, calcium, and iron.

However, teenagers often do not receive important vitamins, minerals, and dietary fiber. They may eat a lot of calories, but from foods high in **saturated fat.** Because teenage males eat more food than teenage females, they are more likely to consume the nutrients they need. Many teenage females fall short in meeting the recommended dietary allowances established by the government.

Teens tend to love foods that are high in fat. However, the increased fat in a teen's diet, especially **unsaturated fat,** may boost the chances of chronic health problems later in life, including obesity. According to the latest statistics from the Centers for Disease Control (CDC), 33 percent of adult men are obese. That means they have a body mass index (BMI) of greater than or equal to 30. In adult women, the obesity rate is 35.3 percent. As for children, 16.3 percent are classified as obese.

Teens and exercise

Diets rich in fat and high in calories as well as a lack of physical activity are impacting the health of America's teens. One of the ways to determine if you are eating a healthy diet is to calculate your BMI. The BMI uses height and weight measurements to determine a specific number, which is then plotted on a chart. By looking at where you fall on that chart, you can tell whether you are underweight, average weight, overweight, or obese.

A BMI of 26 is the cut-off for the definition of obesity in adolescents. According to one study, 23 percent of the teens who participated in the study had a BMI below 19, and 14 percent had a BMI above 26. Fewer than 4 percent had BMIs greater than 30, which is considered extremely obese.

Q & A

Question: What is in a serving?

Answer: According to the federal government's dietary guidelines, a serving fluctuates depending on the type of food being consumed. A serving of cereal is one ounce; a serving of pasta or rice is half a cup; a serving of lettuce is one cup. Knowing the size of a serving will help you understand the nutrition facts label found on packages. More important, knowing what a serving is will make you a healthier person if you abide by those guidelines. If you go to http://mypyramid.gov, you can find specific recommendations just for you.

Boys, girls, and calories

Adolescents need a lot of calories to provide energy for growth and activity. Boys between the ages of 11 and 18 need to consume 2,500 calories each day. Girls in the same age category need only 2,200 calories per day.

Calories come from food. Whether you are a male or a female, calorie intake should be based on the U.S. government's Food Pyramid. There are various representations of the Food Pyramid on boxes and containers of food. The U.S. Department of Agriculture (USDA) first came up with the Food Pyramid in the 1960s. At the time, the Food Pyramid consisted of four food groups. Each food group was stacked on top of another, with the most important food groups located at the wide end of the pyramid. In 2005, however, the USDA added more food groups.

The Food Pyramid sets recommended serving ranges for each of the major food groups. Within those ranges, nutritionists advise teens to choose more or fewer servings based on their consumption of calories.

Most studies show that teenagers do not eat enough fruits, vegetables, and whole grains. The CDC reports that 70.7 percent of all high school students eat fewer than five servings of fruits and vegetables per day. Boys eat only about 4.5 servings of fruits and vegetables per day and also eat less than the recommended daily allowance from the grain food group. Boys tend eat more foods from the meat, cheese, and dairy groups.

Where do teens get most of their calories? More than 33 percent of a teen's daily caloric intake comes from eating snacks between meals. Most snacks, such as potato chips and cookies, are high in fat. Such dietary habits can have terrible consequences. Men are often more at risk from diet-related diseases than women. For example:

- Men are more likely to be stricken with a **cardiovascular** disease than women.
- Men are 1.5 times more likely to die from cancer than women.
- More than two-thirds of all men are overweight or obese.

DID YOU KNOW?

Recommended Servings for Teenagers

Food Group	Number of Servings for Boys	Number of Servings for Girls
Bread, cereal, rice, and pasta	10–11	9
Vegetables	4–5	4
Fruits	3–4	3
Milk, yogurt, and cheese	3	3
Meat, poultry, fish, dry beans, eggs, and nuts	2–3 (about 6–7 ounces)	2 (about 6 ounces)

The chart outlines the number of daily recommended servings in each major food group for both teenage boys and teenage girls.

Source: FamilyEducation.com, 2009.

For their part, women tend to consume less than half the USDA recommendations for vegetables and fruits. However, female teens tend to consume more of the USDA recommendations in the grain and milk group, although the number of servings they consume still falls short. Women also tend to skip breakfast more than men.

Teenage girls need to eat foods that are rich in calcium in order to spur the growth of healthy bone mass. Calcium also reduces the risk of **osteoporosis,** a progressive loss of bone caused by aging. In addition, most nutritionists say that women need double the amount of iron as do men. Most girls do not get their daily supply of iron, and a lack of iron can cause **anemia,** a condition in which a person does not have enough red blood cells and may be tired all the time.

Q & A

Question: Is it better to get your vitamins and minerals from supplements?

Answer: A healthy diet is the best way to get all the vitamins and minerals you need. Food contains a variety of things that supplements do not have, including calories, fiber, and other nutrients. Supplements are designed to supplement your healthy eating habits.

Q & A

Question: I love to snack. How can I control my snacking?

Answer: Ask yourself why you snack. Are you bored, tired, lonely? Is your diet inadequate? If you think about the real reasons for snacking, you may not want to snack on high-fat foods. It is important to eat well-balanced meals and then snack with nutritious foods that are low in fat and high in fiber, such as vegetables and whole grains.

EATING A HEALTHY DIET IS NOT EASY

When you are a teenager, eating healthy foods is sometimes an enormous task. Snacks and junk food are all around you, each day beckoning you to snack and snack more.

It was not that long ago that soda and snack vending machines were a rarity in schools, but not any longer. Many school districts have realized that vending machines are profitable and that they help pay for computers, sports programs, and after-school activities.

Other school districts, realizing the health implications of vending machines, have banned those that sell soft drinks and other junk foods. In addition, the government has stated that school lunches must meet certain guidelines. According to those guidelines, no more than 30 percent of a student's calories should come from fat, and less than 10 percent should come from saturated fat. School lunches are also supposed to supply one-third of the recommended dietary allowances of protein, vitamin A, vitamin C, iron, calcium, and calories.

See also: Body Mass Index; Calories and Weight; Food Groups; Food Pyramid

FURTHER READING

Kirschmann, John. *Nutrition Almanac.* New York: McGraw-Hill, 2006.
Marcus, Bernard A. *Human Nutrition.* Hoboken, N.J.: Cliff Notes, 1997.

■ GROWTH HORMONES

Chemical substances produced to stimulate growth and cell reproduction in humans and animals. Hormones control regular body functions and bring about changes in the functions of various organs according to the body's requirements. Doctors use **synthetic,** or manufactured, hormones to stimulate growth in children and adults who have problems growing normally. In recent years, doctors have treated a number of patients with *human growth hormone* (HGH).

GROWING NORMALLY

If you are a teenager, you are familiar with the term *puberty.* During puberty, the body goes through many changes. Adolescent boys begin puberty between the ages of 10 and 15. For girls, puberty generally begins between the ages of eight and 13. Some teens develop much earlier than their friends; others develop much later.

During puberty, most boys and girls become taller, but some teens may not grow as fast as they should. Sometimes, how tall a person grows depends on that person's **genes,** which contain inherited characteristics, such as eye and hair color. In other words, if your parents are short, chances are that you too will be short. Some teens, however, suffer from a *constitutional growth delay.* In other words, these teens grow normally when they are young, but they do not start puberty until well after their peers. Teens with a constitutional growth delay continue to grow and develop for a few years after all their friends have stopped growing. Generally, these "late bloomers," as they are sometimes called, eventually "catch up" to their friends, usually in their late teens and early 20s.

GROWTH PROBLEMS

There are also teens who have more substantial growth problems. They might have diseases that affect the hormones that control growth. The body's **endocrine system** produces hormones that blood carries throughout the body. Hormones produced by the **hypothalamus,** a part of the brain, control the pituitary gland, which releases hormones responsible for sexual development and growth. Hormones called **estrogen** and **testosterone** also help the body grow.

A condition called *hypothyroidism* can slow a person's growth. The thyroid is a small gland located in the front of the neck that manufactures the hormones that help control growth. To function properly, the thyroid needs **iodine,** a chemical the body absorbs from food. If the thyroid does not produce enough growth hormone, it will diminish a person's ability to grow.

Another cause of slow growth is **dwarfism**. In dwarfs, the body's bones and cartilage grow abnormally, resulting in shorter limbs and shorter body proportions. Another growth disorder is growth hormone deficiency, which begins when the pituitary gland at the base of the brain does not produce the growth hormone needed for normal height. Either the gland does not produce enough of the hormone, or it has completely shut down. There are many reasons why the pituitary gland may not function properly. An accident, trauma, certain diseases, and **tumors** can damage the hypothalamus and impact the growth of the pituitary gland.

GROWTH HORMONE THERAPY

If a physician finds that a person has a lack of growth hormones, he or she might place the patient on a program called growth hormone replacement therapy. The hormone that doctors often prescribe is made in a laboratory, and a patient must take a daily shot of the hormone.

Growth hormone treatment was initially approved by the federal Food and Drug Administration (FDA) for treatment of children who were too short for their age and sex. In order to receive hormone shots, these children had to have a genetic disorder or a growth hormone deficiency. In 2003, the FDA expanded the list of those who could be treated to include kids who did not have any known reason for being short. No one knows the exact numbers of children who receive growth hormone therapy each year.

Does growth hormone replacement therapy work for children who *do not* lack the hormone in their own bodies? The answer seems to be "yes." A recent study by Swedish researchers indicates that growth hormone therapy is effective in children who are not lacking in their natural growth hormones.

The study followed 151 children for 20 years, and researchers concluded that children whose parents were normal in stature responded the best to growth hormone replacement therapy. Those who received higher doses of the hormone grew more than those who received lower doses. A third group received no treatment whatsoever.

Boys who received no treatment grew to an average height of five feet, five inches. Those who got the higher dose grew to a height of five feet, seven inches. Girls who received no treatment reached an average height of four feet, 11 inches. Girls who received the higher dose reached an average height of five feet, two inches.

It can take months before a patient sees the effects of growth hormone replacement therapy. Using the procedure, some children grow an additional two to three inches.

Q & A

Question: I have heard a lot about athletes injecting themselves with human growth hormone. Why do they do that?

Answer: Some athletes believe that HGH gives them a competitive advantage. HGH can increase muscle mass and reduce the amount of body fat in otherwise healthy people. Body builders have long known the effects of HGH. Other athletes, including baseball players, have only recently begun to notice the physical effects of HGH.

HGH creates new muscle cells that remain long after someone has stopped taking the hormone. The longer a person is on the hormone, the more new muscle cells they produce. HGH also strengthens the connective tissues in the body, including *ligaments, tendons,* and cartilage. The result is that old injuries heal quickly, and new injuries can be prevented. HGH also helps the body burn more fat. However, there are serious side-effects with extensive HGH use. A person's facial features, hands, and feet can grow abnormally large. The body's organs and digestive system may also increase in size.

GROWTH HORMONES ON THE FARM

Children and athletes are not the only ones being injected with growth hormones. Many large food producers use growth hormones to boost milk and beef production in cows. Many people, including scientists, are concerned with the effect growth hormones are having on humans.

Most beef and milk packaging does not include a notice that the product comes from animals injected with growth hormones. You do not know whether the beef you are eating or the milk you are drinking came from cows treated with the drug.

Farmers often give their cattle *bovine somatotropin,* or BST, a hormone that interacts with other hormones in the cows' bodies to control the amount of milk they produce. The U.S. cattle industry began injecting cows with hormones in 1956.

See also: Steroids, Anabolic; Weight Training and Weight Management

FURTHER READING

Silverstein Alvin, Virginia Silverstein, and Laura Silverstein. *Growth and Development* (Science Concepts). Minneapolis: Twenty-First Century Books, 2008.

Wilson, Michael R. *The Endocrine System: Hormones, Growth, and Development* (The Library of Sexual Health). New York: Rosen Publishing, 2009.

■ GYMS

Athletic facilities equipped with a variety of physical fitness machines and weights. Some gyms, or fitness centers, have running tracks, racquetball or squash courts, and a pool. Fitness centers are places people go to exercise.

In a gym, there are stair masters, stationary bikes, free weights, rowing machines, universal weights, and treadmills. When you want to work out or when you want to shed some pounds, the local gym is the place to go. In addition to weights and workout machines, many gyms provide a variety of fitness classes, such as **aerobic** workouts. You might have several fitness centers in your hometown. Your school might also have a gym or "weight room" that you can use.

BENEFITS

Gyms provide a place where you can properly balance your exercise routine with a variety of aerobic and **anaerobic** workouts. Aerobic exercises, such as running on a treadmill, are good for the heart and lungs. Anaerobic exercise uses weight training to build muscle strength. Most people join gyms because they do not have the room in their homes for the machines and weights, and such equipment is expensive.

People who join gyms share the equipment with other people. It is much cheaper to join a gym and pay a per-visit or monthly fee than it is to purchase one's own equipment. Most gyms provide access to a personal trainer who can help a client tailor a fitness workout designed specifically for his or her abilities and needs. Most gyms provide a clean, air-conditioned place in which to exercise. Some gyms make working out as convenient as possible. Some are open 24 hours a day, while others offer child-care services, juice bars, saunas, hot tubs, and yoga and Pilates classes. Sometimes, health insurance will help pay for a gym membership. Some businesses have on-site gyms.

Q & A

Question: I'm thinking about joining a gym. What questions should I ask?

Answer: The first question you should ask is simple: Does the gym meet my needs? Why do you want to join a gym? Do you want to lose weight? Do you want to tone up? Are you joining the gym to treat an injury? Does the gym provide the right equipment for your exercise routine? Is the staff qualified? What classes are included with the membership fee? Are there additional charges for these classes? Is the gym clean and well maintained? Look over the equipment. Does it look overused? Are the machines clean? Check out the locker room. Is it clean? What are the membership fees? Do you have to sign a long-term contract? How can you get out of your contract if the need should arise? Does the gym offer discounts for being a student? Can you pay month-to-month? Whatever you do, do not sign the contract right away. Take it home and have someone else read it.

FIRST TIME

Going into a gym for the first time can be a bit stressful. Looking around at all the toned bodies and people working out can sometimes be intimidating. The key for a successful workout experience is to take a new member orientation tour. During the orientation, a trainer will walk around the gym with you describing the benefits of the various machines. Many gyms offer their new customers a health assessment and **body fat** analysis. At no fee, the staff will also show you how to use the weight machines and other equipment.

These sessions are not designed to create a workout regime for you. Instead, the tour is a great way to learn the basics, even if you have worked out before.

GYM LAYOUT

When you first walk into a gym, you will be amazed at the numerous types of machines. One side of the gym might contain fitness machines used for aerobic exercise.

The treadmill is a very popular aerobic machine. Once on the treadmill, a person can either walk or run. One can program, or personalize, the machine's speed and its incline, and treadmills are easy to use.

Elliptical trainers are also very popular. The elliptical machines work like a bike, but instead of pedaling while sitting, one peddles while standing. The stair master, or stair machine, also offers a nice but tough workout. While standing on peddles, one pushes up and down while holding on to handles. The stationary bike is very easy to use, while the stair machine is a little more challenging.

Fact Or Fiction?

Running on a treadmill is better for your joints than running on pavement.

The Facts: Joint pain can occur any time during a workout when pounding any type of surface. While some people can weather the constant pounding better than others, trainers recommend mixing up workouts for the least impact on one's joints. Ease your way into running outside and then run on the treadmill.

Fact Or Fiction?

I'm sore the day after a workout, so I must be doing something right.

The Facts: When you are sore, a number of things can be wrong, none of which has to do with how your muscles are growing. Generally, the pain you feel after a workout comes from inflamed nerve endings and muscle tissue that has been injured. The key is to take it easy at first, and do not push yourself too hard.

Usually on the other side of most gym are machines used for weight training, or anaerobic exercise. Many gyms organize their weight training machines by muscle groups. There are machines for each muscle group, including

- chest press for the chest muscles
- lat pull down for the back muscles
- shoulder press to work out the shoulders
- bicep curl to work out the biceps
- tricep press to work out the triceps
- leg press to work out the various muscles of the lower body, including quadriceps, glutes, and hamstrings

The gym also have leg extension, leg curl, and calf raise machines, not to mention machines for the abdominal muscles. Most gyms also have free weights, which are the traditional dumbbell and barbell weights. If you are a beginner, it might be wise not to use the free weights unless you are familiar with the various exercises you can do with them. Instead, start your workout on the strength machines.

Many gyms offer a variety of classes, including step aerobics, kickboxing, yoga, and Pilates. If you are a bit shy about joining a class, you might want to watch at first. Also, it is sometimes more fun to take a class with a friend.

See also: Aerobic Exercise, Types and Benefits of; Exercise and Strength; Mental Health and Physical Activity; Weight Training and Weight Management

FURTHER READING

Gaede, Katrina, Alan Lachica, and Doug Werner. *Fitness Training for Girls: A Teen Girl's Guide to Resistance Training, Cardiovascular Conditioning and Nutrition.* Chula Vista, Calif.: Tracks Publishing, 2001.
Sharkey, Brian J., and Steven E. Gaskill. *Fitness & Health.* Champaign, Ill.: Human Kinetics, 2007.
Vella, Mark. *Anatomy for Strength and Fitness Training.* London: New Holland Publishers, 2006.

■ INJURIES

See: Exercise and Injuries

■ JOGGING

See: Aerobic Exercise, Types and Benefits of; Carbohydrates and Exercise

■ MENTAL HEALTH AND PHYSICAL ACTIVITY

While researchers and doctors have long known that an increase in exercise promotes better physical health, there is a growing mountain of evidence that physical activity also helps to reduce such psychological health problems as anxiety and depression.

Anxiety disorders are mental conditions that cause biological changes in the brain as a result of feeling excessive fear and dread. Anxiety disorders recur from time to time and are also long-lasting. Depression is also a mental disorder, caused by a chemical imbalance in the brain, in which a person loses interest in activities, has long-lasting feelings of low self-worth, has feelings of guilt, experiences little energy, and has poor concentration. According to the World Health Organization (WHO), depression affects about 121 million people around the world and is the leading cause of disability. Less than 25 percent of those who suffer from depression have access to treatment, according to the WHO. In the United States, depression affects 2 to 5 percent of Americans each year, according to Daniel M. Landers of Arizona State University.

THE RESEARCH

For decades, scientists have suggested that there is a relationship between exercise and a decrease in depression and anxiety. Researchers conducted a number of studies in the 1990s and found that exercise significantly reduced anxiety. In 1996, the Surgeon General of the United States issued a report on physical activity and health. The report stated that "physical activity appears to relieve symptoms of depression and anxiety and improve mood." The report went on to say that "regular physical activity may reduce the risk of developing depression, although further research is needed on this topic."

The research on physical activity and depression goes back to the early 1900s. Researchers suggested in a 1926 study that there was a direct relationship between increased physical activity and a decrease in depression. Through the years, the results consistently showed that there was a direct correlation. Several studies suggested that those who exercise longer and more vigorously have a significant reduction in depression.

Researchers also suggested that anxiety disorders can be reduced through **aerobic** exercise. Aerobic activities include, among other things, walking, tennis, aerobic dancing, jumping rope, and swimming. Unlike anaerobic exercise, aerobic activities are done at a moderate, continuous pace.

The subjects of a 2008 study reported that at least 20 minutes of exercise a week made them feel better mentally than people who did not exercise. The study by British scientists looked at 19,000 men and women in Scotland. Each of the participants filled out a survey about his or her mental health and physical activity. The surveys were taken between 1995 and 2003 and covered myriad activities, including various sports, walking, housework, and gardening. Each of those who participated in the survey answered questions on how often and how hard he or she exercised. The report states that those who were active 20 minutes a week were less likely to suffer various forms of psychological distress than were those who were inactive.

"Although as little as 20 minutes of physical activity might provide some benefit, those individuals that were physically active every day had the lowest risks of mental and physical ill health," researcher Mark Hamer of the University College of London said in an interview with WebMD.com. "Therefore, I'd recommend sticking to current guidelines that suggest at least 30 minutes of moderate to vigorous activity five times per week."

DID YOU KNOW?

Psychological Benefits of Exercise

Confidence   When you are physically active, there is a great sense of accomplishment. No matter how big or small, meeting goals and challenges increases self-confidence, especially when you need it most. Exercise also makes you feel better about the way you look while bolstering self-worth.

Distraction   Exercise literally distracts you from how bad you are feeling. Constantly dwelling on how bad you feel increases the severity of your mental health condition. Exercise shifts the focus from bad feelings to pleasant thoughts.

Interactions   Depression and other mental illnesses can leave a person feeling isolated. Feelings of loneliness can only worsen your condition. Physical activity gives a person a chance to socialize and meet others.

Coping   Exercising is a positive tool and healthy coping strategy.

According to the Mayo Clinic, exercise has many psychological and emotional benefits, especially for people who suffer from anxiety disorders or depression.

Several years ago, researchers at Duke University found that exercise acts as an antidepressant. Other research has shown that exercise improves the brain functions of the elderly and might even protect against **dementia**.

INSIDE THE MIND

In improving mental health, some researchers speculate that exercise activates the production of **endorphins** in the body. Endorphins are natural substances produced by the pituitary gland and the **hypothalamus** that lower pain by reducing the transmission of signals between nerve cells. Researchers speculate that the body produces more endorphins during exercise in response to the natural shock of physical activity. These substances, researchers speculate, improves a person's mood.

Other studies suggest that physical activity causes the brain's frontal lobe to work overtime. Studies in animals found that exercise increases the level of certain **neurotransmitters**, such as **serotonin**, **dopamine**, and **norepinephrine**. Neurotransmitters are chemicals that transmit electrical signals between nerve cells. Scientists also say that exercise increases other substances that improve a person's mood.

A 2001 survey by a British charity called Mind found that 83 percent of people who suffer from mental health problems exercise to feel better. Two-thirds of those who responded said that physical activity helped their mood. More than half said that exercise reduced stress and anxiety. While 50 percent said exercise helped boost **self-esteem**, 60 percent said that exercise helped improve their motivation. Most of those in the survey walked, did housework, or worked in a garden.

TEENS SPEAK

Exercising My Mind

My name is Matt, and I suffer from an anxiety disorder. I can't remember when it all started. I've always been panicky when the new school year starts. How will I do this year? Who will I meet?

Sometimes I have panic attacks and will just pass out with no warning. One time I had a panic attack in gym class. I also became convinced that every time I would step out of the house, something bad would happen. One time I was housebound for a week, until I got up enough nerve to leave.

I was always a shy person. When I was nine, my parents divorced. My mom moved my brother and sister and I to Rhode Island to be near my grandmother. I did not know anyone in Rhode Island. My first day in school was awful. I sat in the corner of the cafeteria the first day. It was a small school, so I stuck out. Some of the kids would snicker behind my back. It was awful.

To make matters worse, my mom remarried. Although he wasn't my dad, I really looked up to him. He was a nice guy, but I still missed my dad. It made me feel sad. We used to do things together, but he was back in California with his new family. The more I thought about it, the more depressed I became. I didn't know why our family had to split up like that. I guess it was one of those things. I started blaming myself, and retreated into my own cocoon. I watched TV or read during most of my free time. I did not have many friends. I was alone. I was sad. I didn't want to be me.

I went to see a doctor. He gave me some medicine. He said it would make me feel better. The pills sort of took the edge off. Then one day, during gym class, Coach Novak ordered us to run around the outdoor track. It was a cool autumn day, just the type of day a person likes to run in. I was never an athlete by any stretch of the imagination. But I was able to run around the track pretty fast. In fact, some of us actually raced. I beat everyone. It made me feel good.

When I got home that day, I did not seem to feel as sad as I used to feel. I couldn't wait to tell my mother that I came in first. She said that I should exercise more if it made me feel good. And that's what I started doing.

Every day after school—or on the days when I didn't have gym class—I ran around the track. I can't describe how I felt in words. I was free, I guess. I didn't worry about my grades, or my family, or anything else. I just focused on running. Soon, I got an iPod and programmed some of my favorite music. Instead of running on the track, my friend Jimmy and I started running on a trail by my house. Jimmy is a better runner than me. We push each other. At first, I used to get winded running up and down the hills. But gradually, I became stronger, and more self-confident.

One time, one of the popular kids in gym class said he could beat me in a race after school. After school one day, we decided to run four laps around the track—that's a mile. A bunch of kids gathered at the stadium that afternoon. The race began, and frankly, I smoked him. We were neck-and-neck for two laps, when I decided to turn my rockets on. I left him in the dust.

Next year, I'm going to join the cross-country team in the fall and the track team in the spring. I think I can do all right. I don't feel as bad as I used to. My doctor says exercising is helping me feel better. I'm glad.

GETTING STARTED

First, check with a doctor. Most mental health specialists encourage exercise as part of the treatment for depression. Talk to your doctor or another health professional, and see how to best go about exercising.

Next, find an activity that you enjoy. If you like to garden or go for a jog, then by all means do it. The key is sticking to an activity.

Set realistic goals. You do not have to run the mile in under four minutes. A 20-minute walk around the block three times a week is a more realistic goal. Once you accomplish that goal, you can set another goal, such as walking around the block in 10 minutes.

Make exercise less of a burden. Some people think that physical activity is a chore. Exercise with a partner. If you do not have a lot of money to spend on fancy exercise equipment or gym memberships, just walk. It's free and simple.

Setbacks will occur, so prepare for those setbacks. If you fail at a achieving a goal, do not worry. Give yourself credit for each step you take. Try again later.

See also: Aerobic Exercise, Types and Benefits of; Exercise and Injuries; Exercise and Strength

FURTHER READING

Cobain, Bev C. *When Nothing Else Matters Anymore: A Survival Guide for Depressed Teens.* Minneapolis: Free Spirit Publishing, 1998.

Johnsgard, Keith. *Conquering Depression and Anxiety Through Exercise.* Amherst, N.Y.: Prometheus Books, 2004.

Moragne, Wendy. *Depression* (Twenty-First Century Medical Library). Minneapolis: Twenty-First Century Books, 2001.

■ METABOLISM

See: Sugar

■ NUTRITIONAL GUIDELINES AND HEALTHY DIETS

Dietary rules published by the federal government every five years to recommend which foods and nutrients should be included in a diet that promotes good health. The guidelines provide Americans, regardless of age, with information about sound nutritional habits. The guidelines are meant to promote good health and reduce the risks for major diseases. The U.S. Department of Agriculture (USDA) issued the last set of guidelines in 2005.

The government's dietary recommendations are based on science. The USDA began providing Americans with dietary guidelines in 1894. The department published its first food guide, "Food for Young Children," in 1916. In 1941, President Franklin Roosevelt called a special National Nutrition Conference to discuss the dietary needs of Americans. Two years later, the USDA issued its first Recommended Dietary Allowance (RDA) standards for Americans to follow. The RDA consisted of five basic food groups, including dairy, grains, proteins, fruits, and vegetables. The RDA outlined the number of servings a person should eat in each of those food groups. In the 1970s, the USDA added a sixth category that included fats, sweets, and alcoholic beverages.

The USDA issued its Food Guide Pyramid to draw attention to the importance of eating healthy foods. The Food Pyramid, as it is commonly called, showed Americans how many servings they should eat from each food group. In 1994, the government began requiring food producers to print nutritional information on their packages. The "Nutrition Facts" labels provide consumers with easy-to-read information on the nutritional content of foods. Because of the guidelines and the Nutrition Facts label, Americans seemingly have no excuse for not knowing how many calories, carbohydrates, and fat they are consuming. One important fact to remember is that the Nutrition Facts label is based on a 2,000-calorie-a-day diet. Some peoples' caloric intake might be higher or lower, depending on the individual.

Reading a Nutrition Facts label is easy. Start with the "Serving Size." The serving size indicates the size of each serving and the number of servings in the package. Serving sizes are usually the same for similar foods.

The next part of the label allows the consumer to check calories and calories from fat. Calories are units of energy. This part of the

Nutrition Facts Label

Nutrition Facts

Serving Size 1 cup (228g)
Servings Per Container 2

Amount Per Serving

Calories 250   Calories from Fat 110

% Daily Value*

Fat 12g	**18%**
Saturated Fat 3g	**15%**
Trans Fat 3g	
Cholesterol 30mg	**10%**
Sodium 470mg	**20%**
Total Carbohydrate 31g	**10%**
Dietary Fiber 0g	**0%**
Sugars 5g	
Protein 5g	

Vitamin A	4%
Vitamin C	2%
Calcium	20%
Iron	4%

* Percent Daily Values are based on a 2,000 calorie diet.
Your Daily Values may be higher or lower depending on
your calorie needs.

	Calories	2,000	2,500
Total Fat	Less than	65g	80g
Sat Fat	Less than	20g	25g
Cholesterol	Less than	300mg	300mg
Sodium	Less than	2,400mg	2,400mg
Total Carbohydrate		300g	375g
Dietary Fiber		25g	30g

This Nutrition Facts label is typical for packages of macaroni and cheese.

Source: U.S. Food and Drug Administration, 2004.

label provides a good indication of how many calories the product has per serving. Counting calories helps consumers manage weight.

The label also indicates the amount of total fat, saturated fat, cholesterol, and sodium, or salt, per serving. On the right side of the label is the percentage of how much of these nutrients you should eat each day. For the example above, a one-cup serving of macaroni and cheese will provide a person with 18 percent of their daily total fat intake. You should consume less of these nutrients.

The next part of the label highlights the nutrients people should be eating to improve health. At the bottom of the label is a food note section with added information about the product.

THE FOOD PYRAMID

The Food Pyramid is another way to inform Americans about dietary needs. The first USDA Food Pyramid consisted of four food groups. Each food group was stacked on top of another depending on how important those foods were to a person's diet. The most important food groups were at the wide end, or base, of the pyramid. The government added more food groups as the years went by.

In 2005, the government replaced its Food Pyramid with a new graphic designed to do a better of job of informing American consumers about their diets. Called MyPyramid, the new food pyramid is less specific than previous ones. The USDA designed the new illustration to depict the variety, moderation, and daily proportions of the six major food groups. The recommendation is that we eat less of the food groups with thinner bands in the pyramid.

In addition to a revamped pyramid, the government issued its last set of Dietary Guidelines in 2005. Those guidelines include the following recommendations, based on a 2,000-calorie diet.

- Eat a variety of foods high in nutrients, while limiting saturated fats, trans fats, alcohol, added sugars, and salt.
- Follow a balanced diet.
- Eat two cups of fruit and two-and-a half cups of vegetables each day.
- Eat at least six ounces of grains a day, with half coming from whole-grain foods.
- Drink three cups of low-fat or fat-free milk each day, or an equivalent of other calcium sources.

■ Limit the total percentage of fat to 20 to 35 percent, with most coming from fish, nuts, vegetable oils, and other unsaturated fats.

■ Choose lean, low-fat, or fat-free proteins.

■ Limit salt intake.

HEALTHY DIETS

According to the Centers for Disease Control and Prevention (CDC), eating right helps you grow, develop, and perform better in school. Eating a healthy diet also prevents health issues, including obesity, eating disorders, dental problems, and **anemia,** which is caused by a lack of iron in a person's diet. Eating healthy foods might also help prevent health problems later in life, including reducing the risk of heart disease, cancer, and stroke–the three leading causes of death.

Remember, eating healthy is not about staying unrealistically thin, or depriving yourself of the foods you enjoy. Instead, eating healthy is more about having more energy, feeling better, and reducing the risks for various illnesses.

The key to a healthy diet is to eat enough calories, but not too many. If you maintain a balance between the calories you consume and the calories you expend through exercise or work, you will be better off. The RDA for calories is 2,000, but this depends on your age, sex, height, weight, and amount of physical activity.

Eating a wide variety of foods, especially whole grains, vegetables, and fruits, is extremely important. Do not overeat. Keep the portions small, especially for foods that are high in calories.

Drink a lot of water. Water helps clean the system of waste products and toxins so that the kidneys and bladder can do their jobs. Limit your intake of sugary foods. For example, just one 12-ounce (340.10 grams) can of soda per day will increase your weight over one year by 16 pounds (7.26 kilograms). Limit your salt, or sodium, intake, too. Exercise regularly.

POOR EATING HABITS

The CDC says that hungry children are more likely to have behavioral, emotional, and academic problems. The CDC also says that poor eating habits and a lack of activity are two of the main reasons that a high percentage of American children are overweight. Many young people suffer from eating disorders. Eating disorders, such as anorexia and bulimia, can cause severe health problems and even death. Nutritional deficiencies in diet and the lack of physical activity cause 300,000 deaths each year in the United States.

In recent years, the diets of Americans have made front-page news, because Americans are getting increasingly fatter. The CDC reports that from 1980 to 2004, the percentage of overweight six to 11 year olds more than doubled, from 7 percent to nearly 19 percent. Moreover, the percentage of overweight 12 to 19 year olds more than tripled, from 5 percent to more than 17 percent, during the same period.

A 2006 study published in the *Journal of the American Medical Association* confirmed that children and adults in the United States are becoming increasingly obese. The study found that between 2003 and 2004, 17.1 percent of all children and adolescents in the United States were overweight. In addition, 32.2 percent of adults were obese. The percentage of overweight female children and adolescents rose from 13.8 percent during 1999–2000 to 16 percent during 2003–04. For that same period, obesity in male children and adolescents rose from 14 percent to 18 percent.

Among men, the prevalence of obesity increased significantly, from 27.5 percent during 1999–2000 to 31.1 percent during 2003–04. Researchers concluded that there was no significant increase in obesity for women between the periods 1999–2000 (33.4 percent) and 2003–04 (33.2 percent).

Approximately 30 percent of white adults were obese, as were 45 percent of black adults. Almost 37 percent of Mexican Americans were obese.

Among adults of all races aged 20 to 39 years, 28.5 percent were obese. Almost 37 percent of adults aged 40 to 59 years were obese, and 31 percent of those aged 60 years or older were obese during 2003–04.

The report summarized that the number of overweight children and adolescents, along with obesity among men, increased significantly during the six-year study period. Women showed no overall increases in the prevalence of obesity.

NUTRITIONAL NEEDS OF TEENS

During the teenage years, the body is growing. Girls experience a growth spurt when they are 10 or 11 years old until they reach about 15. For boys, the growth spurt starts around 12 or 13 and lasts until about 19.

Growth puts stress on the body, especially if a person is not eating the right foods with the right nutrients. Iron and calcium are two nutrients that are extremely important as teenagers grow. Iron supports muscle mass and expands the blood supply. Girls lose iron when they menstruate each month.

Calcium is important for bone growth. Without enough calcium in the diet, a person is at risk for bone loss later in life. The International Food Information Council Foundation says teenagers need about 1,300 milligrams of calcium every day. Studies also show that girls who consume more calcium weighed less and had less **body fat** than girls who did not consume as much. You can get your recommended daily allowance of calcium by eating three servings of dairy products per day. Eating shellfish, broccoli, and leafy green vegetables is another way of getting calcium into your body.

Zinc is another important nutrient for teens. Zinc helps with sexual development and maturation. Various vitamins, such as all of the B vitamins, keep the nerves and blood cells healthy.

See also: Calories and Weight; Dieting and Weight Loss; Food Groups; Food Pyramid; Obesity

FURTHER READING

Dietary Guidelines for Americans, 2005. Washington, D.C.: U.S. Government Printing Office, 2005.

Harris, Dan R. *Diet and Nutrition Sourcebook: Basic Information About Nutrition, Including the Dietary Guidelines for Americans, the Food Guide Pyramid, and Their Applications in Daily Diet* (Health Reference Series). Detroit: Omnigraphics, 1996.

Wardlaw, Gordon M. *Contemporary Nutrition,* 6th ed. New York: McGraw-Hill Science/Engineering/Math, 2005.

■ NUTRITIONAL SUPPLEMENTS

Products such as pills, powders, and drinks that provide additional vitamins or minerals in a person's diet. Also known as dietary supplements, nutritional supplements can also contain herbs and **amino acids.**

A person can purchase dietary supplements from health food stores and drug stores and over the Internet. Doctors sometimes recommend to patients that they supplement their diets with additional vitamins and minerals. Some people take a vitamin or mineral supplement to make sure they get their recommended daily allowance of nutrients every day.

Others, however, use supplements in an attempt to make themselves stronger, slimmer, or smarter or to combat a variety of illnesses.

Dietary supplements have been around for decades. In 1994, the sale of dietary supplements skyrocketed when the U.S. government loosened its regulatory grip on how supplements can be made and sold. At the time, consumer advocates blasted the government for not adequately screening supplements in the same way it screens prescription drugs. The U.S. Food and Drug Administration (FDA) approves all drugs sold in the United States. Before the FDA gives its approval, however, it tests the drugs to make sure they are safe to use.

The FDA does not require that dietary supplements go through the same rigorous testing procedures. Instead, the FDA requires only that the makers of the dietary supplements put a label on their products that reads: "This statement has not been evaluated by the Food and Drug Administration. This product is not intended to diagnose, treat, cure, or prevent disease."

Manufacturers do not have to tell the FDA whether their products are safe or effective. However, the FDA does not allow the producers of dietary supplements to sell unsafe products or products that do not work.

In 2000, however, the FDA further relaxed its rules governing dietary supplements. It said the makers of nutritional supplements can claim to cure certain "passage of life" afflictions, such as acne and morning sickness during pregnancy. The FDA said the manufacturers can make the claims without any proof as to whether the supplement is safe or effective.

Dietary supplements are a $17-billion-a-year business. In fact, the FDA reports that the dietary supplement industry is one of the fastest growing industries in the world.

Fact Or Fiction?

No one is responsible for making sure dietary supplements are safe.

The Facts: Although the FDA does not regulate supplements as carefully it regulates prescription drugs, the manufacturers of nutritional supplements are responsible for making sure their products are safe. However, manufacturers and distributors of supplements are not obligated by law to investigate or tell the FDA of any injuries or illnesses that may be related to or result from the use of their products.

DANGERS OF SUPPLEMENTS

You have seen their claims on television. You have read the advertisements in magazines. Natural memory enhancers and mood boosters are all touted to help you live a better life. Then there are those diet pills that will "just melt the fat away." At lease 50 percent of all Americans take some form of dietary supplements.

However, some people are putting themselves at serious risk. Some supplements may stop the blood from clotting. St. John's Wort, for example, may reduce the effects of birth control pills. Other supplements, such as melatonin, have been linked to seizures in children.

Q & A

Question: How can I tell whether a dietary supplement is safe?

Answer: Because the FDA does not regulate or test dietary supplements, it is up to you to do your homework. The FDA says that you should be suspicious of products that claim to cure a wide range of unrelated diseases. It is foolish to think that one product can cure

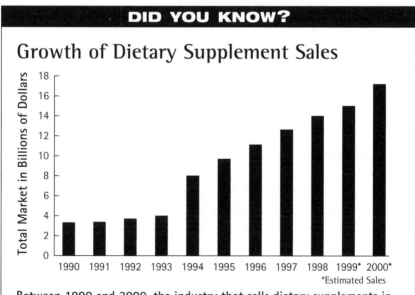

DID YOU KNOW?

Growth of Dietary Supplement Sales

Between 1990 and 2000, the industry that sells dietary supplements in the United States increased its sales dramatically.

Source: Centers for Disease Control and Prevention, 2005.

everything. Also, be wary of ads that suggest a particular product can provide fast and effective relief or a quick cure. If you do not understand the language the manufacturers use to promote their product, stay away from it. Be wary of products that claim "miracle cure," "new discovery," or "magical cure."

Taking too much of a specific supplement, including vitamins and minerals, may cause a *toxic* reaction. Sometimes a person can have a toxic reaction even if they are taking the recommended dose. For example, many people take vitamin C supplements to stave off a cold or to help prevent cancer. Large doses of vitamin C can cause nausea, abdominal cramps, and diarrhea. Excessive amounts of vitamin C can diminish the effect of anticlotting medications.

People who take vitamin B6 supplements in an effort to cure *carpal tunnel syndrome* can cause nerve damage. Some herbs that are used as supplements are also dangerous. They include

- chaparral. This herb may cause hepatitis, a disease of the liver.
- comfrey. Researchers have linked this herb to cancer.
- echinacea. Continual use of echinacea may suppress your immune system, which fights disease.
- kava kava. This herb can damage your *gastrointestinal tract* and discolor your skin, hair, and nails.
- lobelia. Researchers have linked this herb to rapid heart rate, coma, and death.
- yohimbe. This herb has been associated with weakness, paralysis, and death.

In 2003, a pitcher for the Baltimore Orioles baseball team died after taking ephedra, a dietary supplement commonly found in health food stores and drug stores. The makers of the substance advertised ephedra for weight loss and muscle gain. The death of Steve Bechler, 23, was a wakeup call for many who took the supplement. The medical examiner's autopsy cited ephedra as the cause of Bechler's death.

Although the manufacturer of the substance defended the product—they claimed Bechler did not follow the instructions on the label—many health professionals at the time debunked ephedra's promises of long-term weight loss, increased energy, and better athletic performance. They said many people had become ill and even died by taking the supplement.

Two weeks after Bechler's death, federal officials proposed a warning label on the substance stating that it could cause heart attacks, **stroke,** and even death. They also ordered the supplement's manufacturer to stop advertising ephedra as a supplement that builds muscles. In 2004, the FDA banned the substance. Legal challenges to lift the ban proved unsuccessful.

Fact Or Fiction?

The government does not regulate the advertisements for nutritional supplements.

The Facts: The Federal Trade Commission (FTC) is responsible for regulating all the advertising for dietary supplements and other products sold to consumers.

BENEFITS OF SUPPLEMENTS

Not all dietary supplements are bad for you. Many supplements, used correctly, contain much-needed vitamins and minerals that the body uses in small, steady amounts to function properly.

Sometimes people find it difficult to get the recommended daily allowance of vitamins and nutrients they need. Although dietary supplements cannot replace the nutrients found in food, such as fruits and vegetables, they can help.

If you are generally healthy and eat a wide variety of foods such as fruits, vegetables, and whole grains, you probably do not need a dietary supplement. However, if you constantly eat unhealthy foods, or do not eat a variety of foods with the correct amounts of nutrients, dietary supplements might be a good way to get the nutrients your body lacks.

In addition, added vitamins can fight a number of diseases. Sometimes it is not enough to eat healthy foods to correct a vitamin deficiency. Taking supplements is a good idea when a person's energy intake is too low to deliver the needed nutrients to the body's organs.

Those who diet all the time, including vegetarians, may need supplements to stay healthy. The elderly often take supplements because their diets are lacking in specific minerals and vitamins. Sometimes women become anemic during menstruation. An iron supplement can help cure the deficiency, but consult a doctor before taking any supplement.

A calcium supplement might prove beneficial to people who are allergic to milk, or **lactose intolerant.** Calcium is needed for strong bones. Women who are pregnant or breastfeeding their infants need a lot of nutrients, including calcium, iron, and folate, also known as folic acid. Infants also may need supplements. Health care professionals often provide supplements for people being treated for alcohol or drug addictions as well as for patients who suffer a serious injury or have surgery.

Fact Or Fiction?

All ingredients must be printed on the label of a dietary supplement.

The Facts: The FDA does require that certain information, including the ingredients of a dietary supplement, be printed on the supplement's label. Ingredients not listed on the "Supplement Facts" panel must be listed in the "other ingredients" list beneath the panel.

The Mayo Clinic recommends doing the following before you take a vitamin or mineral supplement.

- ■ Read the label. Be sure to read the labels carefully so you know what ingredients and nutrients are included.

- ■ Stay away from supplements that provide "megadoses." Choose a multivitamin-mineral supplement that provides about 100 percent of the Daily Value (DV) of all the vitamins and minerals, rather than one that has, for example, 600 percent of the DV for one vitamin and only 80 percent of the DV for another.

- ■ Check the expiration dates. Dietary supplements can lose their effectiveness over time. Do not buy a supplement if it does not have an expiration date, and throw away all supplements whose expiration dates have expired.

- ■ Store supplements safely. Keep them in a cool place. Keep them out of the bathroom, which can get humid.

- ■ Store supplements out of sight and away from children. Put supplements in a locked cabinet or other secure location.

See also: Gender and Nutrition; Vitamins

FURTHER READING

Hollenstein, Jenna. *Understanding Dietary Supplements* (Understanding Health Series). Oxford, Miss.: University Press of Mississippi, 2007.

Webb, Geoffrey P. *Dietary Supplements and Functional Foods.* Ames, Iowa: Blackwell Publishing, 2006.

■ OBESITY

The condition of having a body mass index (BMI) of 30 or above, meaning body weight is 20 to 30 percent more than a person's ideal weight. Obesity is a **chronic** disease caused by a combination of social, behavioral, cultural, **physiological**, **metabolic**, and **genetic** factors.

To determine whether a person is obese, experts use the body mass index (BMI). A person of healthy weight has a BMI between 18.5 and 25. A person with a BMI between 25 and 30 is overweight. A person with a BMI of 30 or above is obese.

On its most simplistic level, obesity is an excessively high amount of **body fat** in relation to lean body mass. Although there are various methods to determine a person's level of fat, the BMI is the best way. In determining whether a person is obese, experts compare body weight to height.

However, an increase in body fat might not be responsible for someone becoming overweight. A person might simply have an increase in lean muscle. For example, a professional athlete who is lean and muscular with very little body fat might weigh more than a less active person of the same height. Although the athlete is technically "overweight," he or she is not fat.

Obesity is a chronic problem in the United States, one that does not seem to be going away. According to the latest statistics from the Centers for Disease Control and Prevention (CDC), 33 percent of adult men and 35.3 percent of adult women are obese, while 16.3 percent of children are classified as obese. The CDC's 2005–06 National Health and Nutrition Examination Survey was shocking. The CDC found that more than 72 million Americans over the age of 20 were obese. That is a third of the nation's population. In 2006, Americans were twice as likely to be obese as they were in 1980.

The CDC statistics for children are even more disconcerting. Between 1980 and 2004, the number of overweight children and teens tripled, to more than 17 percent. More than 12.5 million young people are currently at risk of various diseases, including diabetes and hypertension, also known as high blood pressure. These are diseases associated with or caused by obesity.

It also appears that Americans are getting fatter at a much younger age than ever before. A study released in 2009 reports that one in five four-year olds are obese. In that age group, obesity is most common in the Hispanic (22 percent) and black (20.8 percent) populations. Those numbers, however, do not compare with the obesity rate for Native Americans, which is an astounding 31.2 percent. The study looked at 8,550 preschool children born in 2001. The survey was conducted by the government's National Center for Education Statistics.

HEALTH PROBLEMS

The health problems associated with obesity are legion. Overweight people often suffer from diabetes, high blood pressure, heart disease, **arthritis**, liver conditions, **stroke**, diabetes, and gout (pain in the joints). An overweight person is also more likely to be at risk for a sleeping disorder called sleep apnea, which occurs when a person's breathing stops periodically for 10 seconds to a minute or more.

In addition, the extra weight carried by people who are obese can damage the body's joints. They may develop osteoarthritis, a degenerative disease of the joints that causes stiffness, inflammation, swelling, and pain.

Cancer and obesity

Researchers also have found mounting evidence that there is a relationship between obesity and cancer. In 2003, the American Cancer Society reported that obesity was responsible for 14 percent of cancer cases in men and 20 percent of cancer cases in women. Researchers followed 900,000 people for 16 years. They concluded that a person has a greater chance of coming down with virtually all types of cancer if he or she is overweight. Men with a BMI of 40 or higher were 52 percent more likely to die from cancer than those with a lower BMI. Women with a BMI of 40 or higher were 62 percent more likely to die from cancer.

In 2002, a report by the American Cancer Society blamed obesity for 41,000 new cases of cancer during that year. Obese women who have gone through **menopause** have 1.5 times the risk of breast cancer than do postmenopausal women of a healthy weight. Obese women have two to four times the risk of developing uterine cancer than do women of healthy weight. Obese men are more likely to suffer from colon cancer than are men of a healthy weight.

Researchers are still examining the links between cancer and obesity. They know that if a person has a high amount of fat tissue, their body produces too much **estrogen** and other **hormones** that impact the way the body's cells work.

Diabetes, heart disease, and other complications

Researchers also say obesity is the main cause of diabetes. In 2006, the CDC reported that people with type 2 diabetes tend to be obese or overweight. Looking at a sample of 31,000 Americans, the CDC researchers found that from 1997 to 2003, there was a 41 percent jump in the number of diagnosed cases of diabetes. In 2003, two of every 1,000 normal-weight people had diabetes. The CDC found during that same year that 18.3 of every 1,000 obese people had diabetes, while 5.5 of every 1,000 overweight people had the disease.

Researchers have also linked obesity with gastroesophageal reflux. This is a condition that causes heartburn when acid from the stomach flows up into the throat.

Obese children are at a greater risk for showing early signs of heart disease, according to researchers at Washington University School of Medicine in St. Louis. "Based on this study, these subtle markers can help us predict who could be at risk for heart disease and heart attacks," said Dr. Angela Sharkey, an associate professor of pediatrics at Washington University School of Medicine.

Researchers looked at data from 168 children between the ages of 10 and 18 who had chest pain, acid reflux, or high **cholesterol.** Scientists determined that 33 of those patients were obese, and 20 were at risk for becoming obese. A total of 115 patients were considered normal. Doctors then looked at the hearts of the obese children with a special imaging machine that tracks movement in the heart muscle's wall. Researchers found that the motion of the heart muscle changed in the obese children. As a child's BMI increased, so did the movement in the heart. Scientists concluded that obese children are more at risk of heart disease than are children with a healthy weight.

Another study presented in 2008 by the American Heart Association found that obese children who have high cholesterol show early signs of heart disease. The study involved 70 children between the ages of six and 19. Researchers found that the thickness of the heart's artery

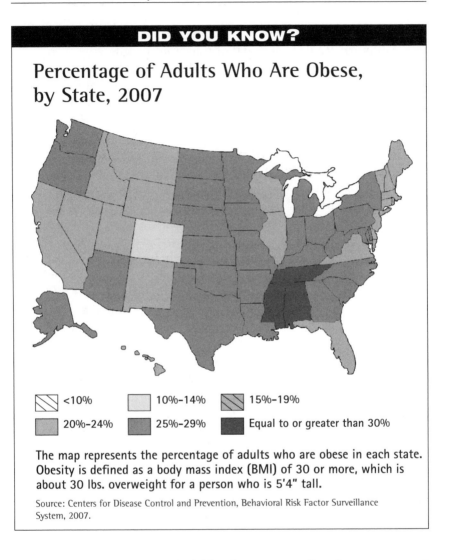

DID YOU KNOW?

Percentage of Adults Who Are Obese, by State, 2007

Legend:
- <10%
- 10%–14%
- 15%–19%
- 20%–24%
- 25%–29%
- Equal to or greater than 30%

The map represents the percentage of adults who are obese in each state. Obesity is defined as a body mass index (BMI) of 30 or more, which is about 30 lbs. overweight for a person who is 5'4" tall.

Source: Centers for Disease Control and Prevention, Behavioral Risk Factor Surveillance System, 2007.

walls in obese children looked like the artery walls of an average 45 year old.

"These findings are potentially consistent with predictions that obesity and its complications would result in cardiovascular disease becoming a pediatric illness," Dr. David Ludwig, an associate professor of pediatrics at Harvard, told the *New York Times.* "This is actually looking at the development of **atherosclerosis,** the process that we know will, if it is not dealt with, lead to heart attack or stroke." Also, in a study of 991 Australian children between the ages of five and 15, researchers found that obese children had enlarged hearts.

WHY ARE AMERICANS OBESE?

Most people are not happy with their weight. How do we gain weight? It's simple. We consume much more energy, or calories, than we burn. Calories are units of energy in food that, when digested in high amounts, lead to weight gain. To gain a pound, you have to eat an extra 3,500 calories without burning those calories off through exercise.

If we consume more calories than we burn, our bodies have to find somewhere to put all that excess energy. The body stores excess energy in the fat cells of our bodies. Obese people have a larger number of fat cells. The cells themselves are also larger. When fat cells reach their maximum size, they divide, creating more fat cells.

Genetics also plays a role in obesity. **Genes** are inherited characteristics, such as eye and hair color. If both parents are obese, there is an 80 percent chance that their children will be obese. When neither parent is obese, there is less than a 10 percent chance that their children will be fat. Genetics also influences the way in which people burn energy.

If a person overeats and does not exercise, he or she will not burn excess calories. As such, that person will gain weight and continue to do so.

Gender also affects the amount of body fat a person has. When girls are young, they have 10 to 15 percent more body fat than boys. Once girls go through puberty, they have 20 to 30 percent more body fat than boys. Boys generally produce more muscle and lean tissue than girls. The extra fat in girls is a normal part of sexual development.

Believe it or not, where someone carries fat can also make a difference. Fat that is stored in the abdominal region is more dangerous to a person's health than fat stored in the hips and thighs. Men tend to store their fat in the abdomen, while women store most of their fat in the hips and thighs. Experts say men with a waistline of more than 40 inches (101.60 centimeters) and women with a waistline of 35 inches (88.90 centimeters) are more likely to experience health problems, such as heart disease and diabetes.

COMBATING OBESITY

There is no magic pill that can help people lose weight. In diagnosing and treating obesity, health care professionals need to assess a person by checking his or her height, weight, and waist size. After the screening, a health care expert can formulate a weight loss plan tailored to an individual's specific needs.

A weight loss diet provides less energy than a person needs to maintain his or her present weight. However, severely restricting energy can do more harm than good. A person should not lose weight too rapidly. Rapid weight loss means a loss of lean tissue. Therefore, the energy intake of an overweight or obese person should be nutritionally sound. Experts say a person should eliminate 10 calories per pound of current weight each day. For example, a 140-pound woman should consume only 1,400 calories a day. As her weight decreases, so should her energy intake. Eating smaller portions and eating more nutrient-dense foods, such as vegetables and fruits, can also help in the battle against the bulge.

Fact Or Fiction?

There is such a thing as a "fat gene."

The Facts: Scientists have studied both humans and animals and have determined that genes play a role in being overweight or obese. At least several dozen genes are involved in obesity, according to the American Dietetic Association. In 1994, scientists found a hormone that fat cells produce. The hormone affects how the body regulates weight and the feeling of being full or not after a meal. The hormone is called leptin. Obese people tend to have an excess amount of leptin in proportion to their BMI. People who suffer from the eating disorder anorexia have low levels of leptin.

It is also important to increase one's activity level to lose weight. Some people have to use extreme measures to lose weight. Many people undergo surgical treatment for obesity, known as bariatric surgery. According to a report released in 2007 from the U.S. Department of Health and Human Services, the number of Americans between the ages of 55 and 64 who underwent bariatric surgery increased from 772 in 1998 to 15,086 in 2004, an increase of 2,000 percent. Children between the ages of 12 and 17 accounted for 349 bariatric surgical cases in 2004. In addition, women have the surgery more often than men.

TEENS SPEAK

My Life Being Overweight

They say that fat people are jolly. That's not true. I am overweight, and I am miserable. My name is Gloria, and I need to lose weight.

If you are reading this, you might think that I'm one of those girls who sits alone in the cafeteria eating potato chips and drinking soda. You might also think that I have no friends. On the contrary, although I am not the most popular girl in school, I have a group of good friends who I hang out with. I'm in the Key Club, the Spanish Club, and I sing in the church choir.

I actually have a lot of fun at school and with my friends. Sometimes, though, I'm embarrassed because I'm overweight. During the summer my friends will often go the beach to hang out. Most of the time, I make up an excuse for why I cannot go. I don't like the way I look in a bathing suit, and I know that other girls and guys stare at me when I walk down the beach. When the Spanish Club has its annual car wash to raise money each May, I'm the only one in the group that doesn't wear a bikini top. And frankly, a lot of guys don't ask me out.

I try to put on a brave face, but my family and friends can see how sad I am. I tried dieting, but I always give in to temptation. I don't have the will power to diet. My mom buys a lot of junk food when she goes grocery shopping. The other day I went to the doctor. I thought she would scold me for being overweight. She didn't. Instead, she urged me to exercise more and change my eating habits. She told me I didn't have to go on a diet, but just change some of the foods I eat. Instead of snacking on cookies, she suggested I munch on carrots, or yogurt. All I had to do was lose 15 pounds to be considered a healthy weight. I'm really going to try. Maybe someday I can walk down the beach and turn heads—this time for all the right reasons.

See also: Calories and Weight; Carbohydrates and Exercise; Food Groups; Food Pyramid; Gender and Nutrition

FURTHER READING

Gay, Kathlyn. *Am I Fat?* Berkeley Heights, N.J.: Enslow Publishers, 2006.

Kaehler, Kathy. *Teenage Fitness: Get Fit, Look Good and Feel Great!* New York: HarperResource, 2001.

■ PROTEINS

Fundamental components of all living cells, including many substances such as **enzymes, hormones,** and **antibodies,** that are essential for the growth and repair of tissue. Proteins are found in meat, fish, eggs, milk and other dairy products, and legumes, such as black beans and lentils. The body's muscles, organs, and immune system are made up mostly of proteins.

One of the six main nutrients found in the human diet, proteins contain the same basic molecular structure as carbohydrates, except that proteins contain nitrogen atoms. The body uses proteins for a variety of tasks, including making **hemoglobin.** Hemoglobin is found in the part of the red blood cells that carries oxygen throughout the body. The body also uses proteins to build up the heart and to fight disease.

AMINO ACIDS

How does protein get into your system? When you eat a juicy steak for dinner, or any other food that contains proteins, the stomach's digestive fluids and the intestines break down the protein into *amino acids*. These fluids include hydrochloric acid and an enzyme called trypsin. Once the amino acids are broken down, the cells of the small intestine absorb the amino acids. The amino acids are then carried to the body's cells. Amino acids are the building blocks of proteins. The body uses amino acids for a variety of things, including maintaining muscles, bones, blood, and organs.

If you could see a protein, you would notice that the **molecules** are long and large, like a string of beads. Each bead has a different shape. Each of those beads is an amino acid. Each bead can band together to make thousands of different proteins. Only 20 amino acids are important to human health. However, the body can make only 11 of those amino acids. They are called *nonessential* amino acids. Nonessential amino acids include

- ■ alanine
- ■ arginine
- ■ asparagine
- ■ aspartic acid
- ■ cysteine
- ■ glutamic acid
- ■ glutamine

- glycine
- proline
- serine
- tyrosine

To form the other nine amino acids, the *essential* amino acids, the body needs help from your diet. Essential amino acids include

- histidine
- isoleucine
- leucine
- lysine
- methionine
- phenylalanine
- threonine
- tryptophan
- valine

Protein from animals, such as meat and milk, contains all nine of the essential amino acids. Proteins from such sources are called *complete proteins*. Vegetables, on the other hand, provide incomplete proteins because they lack one or more of the essential amino acids. For someone who does not eat meat or is allergic to milk, this can present a problem.

Each of the proteins in your body performs a variety of tasks, including

- contributing to enzyme activity that promotes chemical reactions in the body
- telling the body's cells what to do and when to do it
- moving various substances throughout the body
- becoming the building blocks for hormone production
- helping the blood clot
- helping the body fight diseases by promoting antibody activity that controls the immune system

This is a list of several proteins and their functions.

- Antibodies. Antibodies are proteins that protect the body from outside invaders, called antigens. The antibodies stop antigens from moving until the body's white blood cells can come and kill the invaders.

■ Contractile proteins. Every time you raise your hand to answer a question or walk down the hall, contractile proteins are responsible for your body's movement and muscle contractions.

■ Enzymes. Enzymes are often referred to as catalysts because they speed up the various chemical reactions in the body. Lactase and pepsin are two examples of enzymes. Lactase breaks down the sugar in milk. Pepsin works in the stomach to break down proteins in food.

■ Hormonal proteins. Also known as messenger proteins, hormonal proteins help synchronize certain bodily activities. Insulin is an example of a hormonal protein. Insulin regulates the body's ability to metabolize and control **glucose,** or blood sugar.

■ Structural proteins. Structural proteins, such as collagen, elastin, and keratin, are sinewy and provide the body with structural support. Keratins make the hair stronger, while collagen and elastin make the **tendons, ligaments,** and other connective tissue stronger.

■ Storage proteins. Some proteins store amino acids.

■ Transport proteins. Transport proteins are used to move molecules from one place to another. Hemoglobin, for example, moves oxygen through the blood.

PROTEIN DEFICIENCY

If you do not get enough protein in your diet, the consequences could be disastrous. Protein deficiency is rare in developed nations such as the United States, except for those who have poor diets.

In poorer countries, where often there is a low amount of protein in the diet, people sometimes suffer from a disease called kwashiorkor. Among other things, kwashiorkor symptoms include a protruding belly, diarrhea, inability to grow, and peeling skin.

TOO MUCH PROTEIN

Too much protein also can harm the body. A diet high in protein, accounting for more than 30 percent of the daily caloric intake, can damage the kidneys. High-protein diets cause a buildup of ketones, **compounds** produced when the kidneys and liver break down fatty acids. The kidneys work overtime to flush the ketones from the body, causing **dehydration.**

The amount of protein in one's diet is dependent on weight and daily caloric intake. Most Americans consume enough protein in their daily diets.

See also: Dieting and Weight Loss; Food Groups; Food Pyramid

FURTHER READING

Royston, Angela. *Proteins for a Healthy Body.* Chicago: Heinemann, 2009.
Centers for Disease Control and Prevention. "Nutrition for Everyone: Protein." Available online. URL: http://www.cdc.gov/nutrition/everyone/basics/protein.html. Accessed April 23, 2010.

■ RUNNING

See: Aerobic Exercise, Types and Benefits of; Carbohydrates and Exercise

■ SALT (SODIUM) AND WATER BALANCE

The relationship, or balance, maintained by the body between the amount of water in the body and the amount of mineral salts, such as sodium. When sodium, known as an **electrolyte,** becomes too high, a person gets thirsty, leading to an increase in the intake of fluids. As such, the body's kidneys expel less urine. As a person drinks more liquid, the bloodstream becomes awash in water, diluting the body's sodium content. When that happens, the body's salt-to-water balance is restored.

When the amount of sodium in the body becomes too low, the kidneys emit more urine, which decreases the amount of water in the bloodstream. This process restores the balance between sodium and water.

WATER AND YOU

If you were to look inside the body, you would see organs, **veins,** and **arteries.** You would also see lots and lots of water, because, in fact, the human body is 65 percent water. A person needs to drink eight to 10 cups of water a day to replenish what the body loses.

Water is the human body's most important nutrient. One can live weeks, or even months, without food, but someone would survive only eight to 10 days without water. Water moves through our body via the bloodstream and **lymphatic system** and transports oxygen and nutrients to the body's cells. The body also uses water to remove waste through urine and sweat and to maintain a healthy balance between dissolved salts, such as sodium.

A half to two-thirds of human weight is made up of water. The amount of water in an average woman is less than in an average man. Water makes up 52 to 55 percent of a woman's body, while the average male consists of about 60 percent. The percentage of water is less in an elderly person, while an obese person has a higher percentage of water. Water makes up about 70 percent of a newborn child's body.

If your father or uncle weighs 150 pounds (68 kilograms), he will have about 10 gallons (38 liters) of water in his body. Where is all that water located? Six to seven gallons (23 to 27 liters) of water can be found inside the body's cells. Two gallons (7 liters) of water take up the space around the cells. Only about one gallon (4 liters) of water is located in the bloodstream.

The body ensures that the amount of water in each of these areas is constant. That helps the body function normally. You must refill your body with water quickly when you lose it. Experts recommend drinking one and a half to two quarts (2 liters) of fluids a day. If you dehydrate, or lose water, you can develop a number of medical problems, including kidney stones. Drinking too much water is better than not drinking enough. Your body will automatically dispose of excess water.

The body's cells and tissues obtain water through the digestive process. In addition, your body produces some water when it **metabolizes** various nutrients. The body expels water through the kidneys by disposing of it via urine. A person can pass a pint to several gallons of urine a day, depending on the individual. The body also loses excess water through perspiration and through the lungs. People can also lose water if they vomit or have prolonged diarrhea. If these health issues are severe, a person can dehydrate.

SODIUM

Sodium is a chemical element found in table salt, which is made from **molecules** of sodium and chloride. Salt is essential for normal nerve

The Minerals We Need

Mineral	Good Sources	Main Functions	Recommended Dietary Allowance	Safe Upper Limit
Calcium	Milk and milk products, meat, fish eaten with the bones (such as sardines), eggs, fortified cereal products, beans, fruits, and vegetables	Required for the formation of bone and teeth, for blood clotting, for normal muscle function, for the normal functioning of many enzymes, and for normal heart rhythm	1,000–1,200 mg for people over 50	2,500 mg
Chloride	Salt, beef, pork, sardines, cheese, green olives, cornbread, potato chips, sauerkraut, and processed or canned foods (usually as salt)	Involved in electrolyte balance	1,000 mg	—
Chromium	Liver, processed meats, whole-grain cereals, and nuts	Enables insulin to function (insulin controls blood sugar levels); helps in the processing (metabolism) and storage of carbohydrates protein, and fat	35 mcg for men aged 50 and younger; 25 mcg for women aged 50 and younger; 30 mcg for men over 50; 20 mcgs for women over 50	—

(continues)

DID YOU KNOW? (CONTINUED)

Copper	Organ meats, shellfish, cocoa, mushrooms, nuts, dried legumes, dried fruits, peas, tomato products, and whole-grain cereals	A component of many enzymes that are necessary for energy production and for formation of the hormone epinephrine, red blood cells, bone, and connective tissue	900 mcg	10,000 mcg
Fluoride	Seafood, tea, and fluoridated water	Required for the formation of bone and teeth	3 mg for women; 4 mg for men	10 mg
Iodine	Seafood, iodized salt, eggs, cheese, and drinking water (in amounts that vary by the iodine content of local soil)	Required for the formation of thyroid hormones	150 mcg	1,100 mcg
Iron	Beef, poultry, fish, kidneys, liver, soybean flour, beans, molasses, spinach, clams, and fortified grains and cereals	Required for the formation of many enzymes in the body; also an important component of muscle cells and of hemoglobin, which enables red blood cells to carry oxygen and deliver it to the body's tissues	8 mg for women over 50 and for men; 18 mg for women aged 50 and younger; 27 mg for pregnant women; 9 mg for breast-feeding women	45 mg

Magnesium	Leafy green vegetables, nuts, cereal grains, beans, and tomato paste	Required for the formation of bone and teeth, for normal nerve and muscle function, and for the activation of enzymes	320 mg for women; 420 mg for men	—
Manganese	Whole-grain cereals, pineapple, nuts, tea, beans, and tomato paste	Required for the formation of bone and the formation and activation of certain enzymes	2.3 mg for men; 1.8 mg for women	6 to 11 mg
Molybdenum	Milk, legumes, whole-grain breads and cereals, and dark green vegetables	Required for metabolism of nitrogen, the activation of certain enzymes, and normal cell function; helps break down sulfites (present in foods naturally and added as preservatives)	45 mcg	1,100 to 2,000 mcg

(continues)

DID YOU KNOW? (CONTINUED)

Phosphorus	Dairy products, meat, poultry, fish, cereals, nuts, and legumes	Required for the formation of bone and teeth and for energy production; used to form nucleic acids, including DNA (deoxyribonucleic acid)	700 mg	4,000 mg
Potassium	Whole and skim milk, bananas, tomatoes, oranges, melons, potatoes, sweet potatoes, prunes, raisins, spinach, turnip greens, collard greens, kale, other green leafy vegetables, most peas and beans, and salt substitutes (potassium chloride)	Required for normal nerve and muscle function; involved in electrolyte balance	3.5 g	—
Selenium	Meats, seafood, nuts, and cereals (depending on the selenium content of soil where grains were grown)	Acts as an antioxidant, with vitamin E; required for thyroid gland function	55 mcg	400 mcg

DID YOU KNOW? (CONTINUED)

	Sources	Function		
Sodium	Salt, beef, pork, sardines, cheese, green olives, corn bread, potato chips, sauerkraut, and processed or canned foods (usually as salt)	Required for normal nerve and muscle function; helps the body maintain a normal electrolyte and fluid balance	1,000 mg	2,400 mg
Zinc	Meat, liver, oysters, seafood, peanuts, fortified cereals, and whole grains (depending on the zinc content of soil where grains were grown)	Used to form many enzymes and insulin; required for healthy skin, healing of wounds, and growth	15 mg	—

G=grams; mg=milligrams; mcg=micrograms.

By measuring the levels of minerals in a person's blood or urine, physicians can detect many health problems, including an electrolyte imbalance. The chart lists the minerals the body needs, what they are used for, and the Recommended Dietary Allowance for adults.

Source: Merck Manuals Online Medical Library, 2008.

and muscle function. As an electrolyte, salt and other substances, such as **potassium,** allow the kidneys to regulate the body's fluid levels. The body also uses electrolytes to maintain the correct acid-base balance.

The body needs to keep its fluid levels from varying too much if it is to remain healthy. That means there has to be sufficient fluid within the body's cells, around the body's cells, and in the bloodstream. Having electrolytes, such as sodium, in the right balance is essential for good health. The body transports electrolytes into and out of cells. The kidneys maintain the electrolyte balance by filtering the substances from the blood and returning some electrolytes to the body's cells. If the balance between water, sodium, and other electrolytes is thrown off, a person can become dehydrated or have heart, kidney, or liver problems.

BALANCING ACT

Thirst is the primary method by which the body maintains its balance of water and sodium. Certain parts of the brain are stimulated when the body needs water. As a result, people develop thirst. A person gets more thirsty as the body's need for water increases. When you have quenched your thirst, the brain is no longer stimulated. As such, you do not have a desire to drink more fluids.

When you are low on water, the body's pituitary gland, located at the base of the brain, produces a **hormone** called *vasopressin.* The pituitary gland releases the hormone into the blood stream, which then tells the kidneys to release less urine and conserve water. When the body has too much water, the pituitary gland produces less vasopressin. That allows the kidneys to release excess water in the urine.

FORCED DEHYDRATION IN ATHLETES

Dehydration occurs when the body uses more fluids than it takes in. Dehydration can occur for various reasons, including illness, prolonged exposure to high temperatures, or simply not drinking enough water. Dehydration upsets the body's balance of salt and water.

Many athletes, including boxers and wrestlers, however, often force themselves to dehydrate to lose weight quickly in order to make their weight classifications before competitions. Athletes normally do this by cutting back on liquids or through excessive exercise before the "weigh-in." Other techniques of forced dehydration include use of **diuretics, laxatives,** spitting, and bloodletting. Wrestlers often use saunas or rubber suits in order to sweat out fluids so they can make weight.

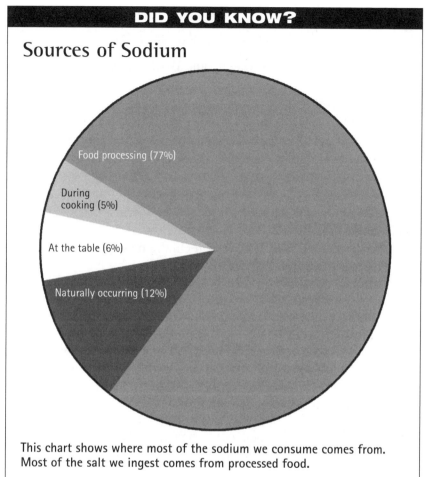

Sources of Sodium

This chart shows where most of the sodium we consume comes from. Most of the salt we ingest comes from processed food.

Source: U.S. Department of Agriculture, 2008.

CHRONIC DEHYDRATION

Anyone can become dehydrated for any number of reasons. If the body is not getting enough fluids, the impact on a person's health can be dangerous. Some of the symptoms of chronic dehydration include a dry or sticky mouth, low or no urine output, the inability to produce tears, and lethargy.

Chronic dehydration takes time to correct. Drinking one or two glasses of water will not help. Sometimes hospitalization is necessary. While in the hospital, doctors begin a course of intravenous fluid replacement. Chronic dehydration can also lead to organ failure, diabetes, eating disorders, lung disease, and kidney disease.

See also: Anorexia Nervosa; Dieting and Weight Loss; Eating Disorders

FURTHER READING
Batmanghelidj, Fereydoon. *You're Not Sick, You're Thirsty! Water for Health, for Healing, for Life.* New York: Warner Books, 2003.
——. *Your Body's Many Cries for Water.* Vienna, Va.: Global Health Solutions, 1995.

■ SKIN CANCER

Abnormal growth of skin cells caused chiefly by exposure to the sun. People spend hours tanning their bodies, either by lying in the sun or going to tanning salons. Those who are tanned are automatically assumed to be physically fit. A tanned body radiates a perception of health, vigor, and vitality. Many professional gyms offer customers the use of tanning booths.

However, exposure to ultraviolet (UV) light, either from the Sun or tanning booths, can lead to skin cancer, one of the most common forms of cancer. Skin cancer can be avoided by limiting exposure to UV rays. It is also important to monitor any changes on the skin.

According to the National Cancer Institute, there were more than 1 million new cases of skin cancer in 2008 and 1,000 deaths. The three main types of skin cancer include

- Basal-cell carcinoma. Basal-cell carcinoma forms in the small round cells in the base of the outer layer of the skin. This type of cancer grows slowly on areas of the skin that have been exposed to the sun.

- Squamous-cell carcinoma. This type of cancer forms in flat cells on the surface of the skin. Exposure to the sun is not a precondition for squamous-cell skin cancer. Squamous-cell cancer can sometimes spread to the body's **lymph nodes** and organs.

- Melanoma. Melanoma is the most serious type of skin cancer. It forms in the skin cells that determine a person's pigment. More than 53,600 people in the United States learn each year that they have melanoma. The percentage of people who have developed this particular form of skin cancer has doubled in 30 years. Malignant melanoma claims an estimated 8,000 lives each year in the United States. It is the most common cancer in young women aged 25 to 29, according to recent studies. Repeated sunburns and habitual exposure to strong sunlight increases the risk for developing the disease.

WHAT IS SKIN?

The skin is the largest organ of the human body. It protects against light, heat, injury, and infection. The skin is waterproof and helps control the body's temperature. It is made up of two major layers. The first layer is the *epidermis,* the top layer of skin. The epidermis is made up of flat cells called *squamous* cells. Deeper into the epidermis is a layer of round cells called *basal* cells. At the very bottom of the epidermis are *melanocytes,* the cells that give the skin its color, or pigment.

The second major layer of the skin is the *dermis.* The dermis is directly under the epidermis and contains blood vessels and the glands that produce sweat. Sweating is the way the body cools itself. The dermis is also home to other glands that keep the skin from drying out.

WHAT IS CANCER?

Any type of cancer is caused by **mutations,** or changes, in a cell's DNA. DNA is the abbreviation for the genetic material **deoxyribonucleic acid. Genes** determine inherited characteristics, such as eye and hair color. Exposure to a wide variety of conditions in the environment can cause a cell to mutate.

A normal cell grows and divides into new cells. When someone suffers from skin cancer, something inside the cell goes horribly wrong. New cells form when they should not, and old cells do not die when they should. Eventually, these extra cells form a **tumor.** Tumors are often benign, that is, not life-threatening, and can easily be removed. Benign cells do not spread to other parts of the body.

On the other hand, malignant cells can cause death. Surgeons can remove malignant cells, but they sometimes grow back and spread to other parts of the body.

RISKS

Some people are more likely than others to develop skin cancer. Studies have found that one of the main causes is exposure to UV radiation. UV radiation comes from the Sun. UV also comes from sunlamps, tanning beds, and tanning booths. People with fair skin or freckles and those who sunburn easily are at a greater risk for developing skin cancer than others.

In addition, skin cancer rates are greatest in warm climates. People who live in certain regions of the country, such as the South and the Southwest, are more likely to be exposed to the Sun's harmful rays than those living in Maine or Michigan. Moreover, it does not have to be warm outside to be exposed to UV rays. UV rays beam down from the Sun during cool, clear, sunny, winter days. Even people who live in the mountains are more likely to suffer from skin cancer than those living at lower-altitudes.

Fact Or Fiction?

One application of sunscreen a day can protect me from skin cancer.

The Facts: Using sunscreen when you are outdoors is always a good idea. However, you need to reapply the sunscreen continuously, and even then it offers only a limited amount of protection. The best way to make sure you are protected from UV rays is to cover up as much skin as possible. In addition, use sunscreen with an SPF, or sun protection factor, of 15 or higher. Wear a hat that shields your face, neck, and ears. Wear sunglasses. Stay out of the sun between 10 A.M. and 4 P.M., when the Sun's rays are the strongest.

Fact Or Fiction?

Only fair-skinned people can get skin cancer.

The Facts: Not so! African Americans, Asians, and others who are dark skinned can also get skin cancer. Many times the cancer will show up under the fingernails or on the soles of the feet.

Fact Or Fiction?

Lip gloss can protect the skin of my lips.

The Facts: Scientists at Baylor University Medical Center in Dallas, Texas, found that lip balms and glosses actually attract UV rays, raising your risk of skin cancer.

DID YOU KNOW?

Estimated U.S. Cancer Cases for 2009

	Men 766,130	Women 713,220	
Prostate	25%	27%	Breast
Lung & bronchitis	15%	14%	Lung & bronchus
Colon & rectum	10%	10%	Colon & rectum
Urinary bladder	7%	6%	Uterine corpus
Melanoma of skin	5%	4%	Non-Hodgkin lymphoma
Non-Hodgkin lymphoma	5%	4%	Melanoma of skin
Kidney & renal pelvis	5%	4%	Thyroid
Leukemia	3%	3%	Kidney & renal pelvis
Oral cavity	3%	3%	Ovary
Pancreas	3%	3%	Pancreas
All other sites	19%	22%	All other sites

According to projections by the American Cancer Society, skin cancer will account for 5 percent of all the estimated cancer cases for men and 4 percent of all estimated cancer cases for women in the United States in 2009.

Source: American Cancer Society,2009.

TANNING SALONS

Those who frequent tanning salons are putting themselves at risk for skin cancer. The World Health Organization, the American Medical Association, and the American Academy of Dermatology all report that tanning salons are just as dangerous to a person's health as cigarettes. Since 2003, 19 states have banned anyone under 18 from using a tanning salon. With more recent reports of the danger, those bans will likely increase.

The science on just how tanning salons relate to the growing rates of skin cancer is ambiguous, at best. In 2002, the U.S. government conducted a study on the hazards of UV radiation coming from the Sun or other sources. That study concluded that UV radiation, no matter what the source, causes skin cancer. Although another government study by the Food and Drug Administration had reported that the evidence that UV rays cause skin cancer was inconclusive, scientists reported in 2009, that the risk of getting skin cancer increased by 75 percent when people begin using tanning beds before they turn 30.

The tanning salon industry reports that 30 million people each year safely use tanning beds and booths. The American Cancer Institute says that everyone who uses tanning booths or tanning beds is putting themselves at risk for skin cancer. The Cancer Institute says that tanning can be extremely dangerous for people who are fair-skinned or who have red or light-colored hair. Tanning is also dangerous for those who burn easily.

TEENS SPEAK

My Skin Cancer

My name is Jane, and I used to spend a lot of time outside. I lived in the country. If I was not swimming at the lake, or hiking one of the many trails near my home, I was helping my dad outside. I enjoyed the outdoors and would always have a nice healthy tan because I was outside all of the time.

A couple of years ago, dad got sick. So we had to move to the city to stay with my grandmother. I missed being tan and out in the sun. One day at school, my new friend, Jennifer, told me about the tanning salon she went to. She asked me to go with her. I did. Little did I know that when I was outside all of the time, my skin was damaged by the sun. That, coupled by frequent trips to the tanning salon, caused me to get skin cancer on my shoulders. At first, I thought the sore was a bite or a scrape of some type. But it kept growing and growing.

Finally, I went to the doctor. He took a small sample and a few days later called me up with the bad news—I had skin cancer. He removed the lesion. The cancer has not returned. Today, I stay away from tanning salons. When I'm outside I slather sun block on my body. I use SPF 30. I always check for lesions or sores. I'm glad I caught the cancer in time.

TREATMENT

Getting skin cancer is not an automatic death sentence. If detected early, most basal-cell and squamous-cell cancers can be cured. The key is to watch out for any changes on the skin, such as small, smooth, shiny, pale, or waxy lumps; a firm red lump; or a sore or lump that bleeds or develops a scab.

Once you find something that you think is abnormal, it is the job of a doctor to determine whether the lump is cancerous. Doctors often perform a **biopsy** to determine if cancer is present. The doctor will take a small sample and have a **pathologist** look at the cells to determine if they are cancerous.

Sometimes the doctor will remove all of the cancer during the biopsy. If that occurs, no other treatment is necessary. Of course, treating skin cancer depends on the type of cancer and what stage it is in. Where the cancer is located on your body, along with your previous medical history, also determine the treatment options. Sometimes doctors need to perform surgery to cut out the cancer. Other times, doctors prescribe anticancer drugs to kill the cancer. Most of the time, the drugs come in the form of a lotion and need to be applied two or three times a day for several weeks.

Another way to treat skin cancer is with photodynamic therapy (PDT). PDT uses a chemical and a laser to kill the cancer cells. The doctor injects the chemical into the cancer cells, then focuses a laser light on the cells. The chemical becomes active and kills the cancer cells. Treating cancer with radiation is another treatment option for skin cancer, although very uncommon.

FURTHER READING

Barrow, Mary Mills, and John F. Barrow. *Sun Protection for Life: Your Guide to a Lifetime of Healthy & Beautiful Skin*. Oakland, Calif.: New Harbinger Publications, 2005.

Juettner, Bonnie. *Skin Cancer* (Diseases and Disorders). Farmington Hills, Mich.: Lucent Books, 2007.

So, Po-lin. *Skin Cancer* (The Biology of Cancer). New York: Chelsea House, 2007.

■ SLEEP AND PHYSICAL FITNESS

Sleep is one of the cornerstones of being physically fit. At the same time, the amount of physical exercise one gets during the day also determines how good one's sleep is at night. Once a person starts on an exercise program, the quality of sleep is greatly improved. Research underscores the direct correlation between how much people exercise and how they feel afterward. Sleep and exercise can make you more alert, speed up your **metabolism,** and give you a lot of energy for the day ahead.

Conversely, lack of sleep can cause a myriad of health problems. In fact, lack of sleep is a vicious cycle. The less time you sleep, the more tired you are. The more tired you are, the less active you are. The less active you are, the more health problems you have. Studies have even linked lack of sleep to heart disease and diabetes. Researchers in London found that lack of sleep can double a person's chances for heart disease, weight gain, and high blood pressure. In addition, chronic sleep loss is tied to obesity.

SLEEP TIGHT

Many species of animals, including humans, need sleep to survive. The National Sleep Foundation recommends that people sleep six to seven hours each night. A study by researchers at the University of California, San Diego, found that people who live the longest sleep more than seven to eight hours a day. Children need more sleep than adults, up to 18 hours for newborn babies.

In teenagers, a good night's sleep is important. Teens need about 9.25 hours of sleep each night. However, most teens do not get that amount of sleep. They typically stay up late and sleep late on the weekends. Lack of sleep makes teenagers more prone to getting acne and being impatient with family and friends.

Getting a good night's sleep is not as easy as it seems. About 18 million Americans suffer from sleep apnea, a disorder in which a person stops breathing repeatedly while asleep. Not only can sleep apnea ruin a good night's sleep, it also can lead to **stroke**, heart attack, congestive heart failure, and general tiredness during the day. Most people who have been diagnosed with sleep apnea are generally overweight.

Some 50 to 70 million Americans suffer from chronic sleep disorders, according to the National Institutes of Health. Insomnia, the inability to fall and remain asleep, can last for a night or for years. According to the National Center for Sleep Disorders Research and the National Institutes of Health, about 30 to 40 percent of adults say they have experienced insomnia.

Q & A

Question: What role does sleep have in a person's risk of developing type 2 diabetes?

Answer: According to a six-year study, people who slept less than six hours a night were likely to develop a condition that precedes the onset of diabetes. A team of researchers at the University of Buffalo, in New York State, said those who slept less than six hours a night during the week were 4.56 times more likely to develop a condition called impaired fasting glucose than those who slept six to eight hours. The condition arises when blood sugar levels become too high, but not high enough to warrant a diagnosis of diabetes.

SLEEP AND EXERCISE

The National Sleep Foundation reports that exercising in the afternoon can help a person cut down on the amount of time it takes to fall asleep. However, exercising too much before bedtime can have the reverse effect.

In 2003, researchers at the Fred Hutchinson Cancer Research Center concluded that exercise helps people sleep better at night. Researchers said that **postmenopausal** women who exercised 30 minutes every morning had fewer problems falling asleep than women who were less active. Those who worked out in the evening saw little or no improvement in their sleep patterns.

Another report from Stanford University Medical Center concluded that older and middle-aged people who exercised routinely reported better sleep habits. In setting up the study, researchers selected 29 women and 14 men aged 50 to 74. All of the participants in the study complained of mild sleep problems and lived fairly sedentary, or inactive, lives. They had no symptoms of heart disease, stroke, or any known sleep disorder. All were nonsmokers and occasional drinkers of alcoholic beverages.

Researchers had the men and women exercise four times a week. They took an aerobic class twice a week, which included 30 minutes of strength and endurance exercises. They also rode a stationary bike or took a walk twice a week for 40 minutes. The subjects who exercised moderately during the 16-week trial were able to fall asleep 15 minutes sooner and slept about 45 minutes longer at night than before, the researchers reported.

See also: Aerobic Exercise, Types and Benefits of; Disease and Inactivity; Exercise and Injuries; Exercise and Strength

FURTHER READING

Bean, Dianne. *Nutrition Ambition.* Orlando: Bauz Publishing, 2007.
Thayer, Robert E. *Calm Energy: How People Regulate Mood with Food and Exercise.* New York: Oxford University Press, 2001.

■ SODIUM
See: Salt (Sodium) and Water Balance

■ SPORTS DRINKS AND ENERGY BARS
Products designed to provide energy and nutrition during exercise. Sports drinks, such as Gatorade, are manufactured to help athletes hydrate themselves during physical activities. Sports drinks are used to replace **electrolytes**, carbohydrates, and other nutrients lost during exercise or competition. Replacing electrolytes is important in hydrating the body and reducing fatigue. The drinks also replace the carbohydrates the body burns during exercise.

Some energy bars, such as PowerBar, are high in carbohydrates and low in fats. They are made mostly of high-fructose corn syrup, vitamins and minerals, and other ingredients.

The sale of sports drinks and energy bars is a big business in the United States. According to one report, the sports food and drink industry grew 48 percent between 2000 and 2005, reaching sales of $6.1 billion a year. Some sports drinks and energy bars promise to increase energy levels and alertness. Others offer extra nutrition, while some promise to increase concentration or better athletic performance.

HYDRATION NATION
Whether hiking on the Appalachian Trial, running a marathon, or playing a blistering game of tennis, keeping the body hydrated during physical activity is important. During exercise, the body loses fluids rather quickly. **Dehydration** sets in when the body uses more fluids than it takes in. The body uses electrolytes to maintain the correct acid-base balance.

If the body is to function properly, it must prevent fluid levels from fluctuating wildly. That means there has to be sufficient fluid within the body's cells, around the body's cells, and in the bloodstream. Having electrolytes, such as **potassium**, in the right balance is essential during exercise. A person can become dehydrated when the balance between water, sodium, and other electrolytes is thrown off.

One way of maintaining that balance during exercise is to drink liquids. Many people choose to consume sports drinks. Although sports drinks can help you get through a vigorous round of exercise and might help to keep your electrolytes in balance, the infusion of carbohydrates is what actually makes sports drinks valuable.

Carbohydrates are chemical **compounds** containing carbon, hydrogen, and oxygen. The simplest carbohydrates are sugars, such as **glucose** and fructose. When you eat, your body's digestive system converts these carbohydrates to glucose. Your body turns some glucose into energy and also stores some glucose in the liver and muscles.

Glycogen is the source of energy the body uses during exercise. Glycogen supplies energy during prolonged physical activity, such as running or swimming laps in a pool. If there is not enough glycogen in a person's system during exercise, he or she will become tired fairly quickly. If a person is fatigued, the ability to continue to exercise or compete becomes limited. The ingredients of most sports drinks include water, sugar, sodium, potassium, corn syrup, and fructose.

Sports drinks are also high in calories. Excess calories are good for athletes who burn a lot of calories in high-impact sports such as competitive cycling and running a marathon. However, if you are an armchair quarterback, you might want to reduce your intake of these fluids. A person's body does not need the added sugar and calories, which contribute to weight gain. If you are trying to lose weight and are using sports drinks, you should cut down on the amount of calories you consume elsewhere in your diet. As for the boost of electrolytes these sports drink give, a report in the journal *Sports Medicine* said that electrolytes, such as sodium and potassium, will not do you any good unless you sweat continuously for four hours.

Energy drinks are also packed with caffeine. Caffeine is a stimulant and can cause a variety of problems, including stomachaches, headaches, and sleep problems.

Q & A

Question: Which is a better way to rehydrate during exercise, drinking water or drinking a sports beverage?

Answer: Research shows that when a teenager or child exercises vigorously for an hour, water is just as good as sports drinks. Water not only rehydrates a person, it keeps the electrolytes in balance. Water also doesn't increase the level of sugar in the body and contains no calories.

TOOTH DECAY

While sports drinks rehydrate after a workout, if you consume vast amounts of these liquids, you could be setting yourself up for dental problems later on. A study presented in 2009 at the International Association for Dental Research concluded that sports drinks, such as Gatorade, PowerAde, and Life Water, can damage tooth enamel. Mark Wolff, a professor at New York University College of Dentistry, and his associates looked at the way sports drinks affected **dentin,** the tissue under the enamel that determines what teeth look like and how large they get.

The scientists soaked cow teeth, which are similar to human teeth, in several top-selling sports drinks for 75 to 90 minutes. Afterward, researchers measured how strong the teeth were. Since sports drinks have a high acid content, they weakened the enamel. Enamel protects teeth from bacteria. When the enamel is weakened, it gives bacteria a chance to grow in the cracks of the teeth. Sugar, a major ingredient in sports drinks, exacerbates this because bacteria feed off sugar. The combination of acid and sugar is lethal to a tooth, causing it to decay.

Wolff recommends that people should not consume sports drinks as their beverage of choice every day. However, a study by Ohio State University concluded there is no relationship between tooth decay and sports drinks.

BRAIN DRINK?

Also in 2009, a study published in the *Journal of Physiology* concluded that energy drinks may boost performance during exercise. Researchers say that people may have areas in the mouth that are sensitive to carbohydrates. The carbs activate those areas in the mouth, which then send a message to the brain, thereby boosting an athlete's performance.

The study used a group of cyclists. Researchers asked the cyclists to compete in a vigorous workout. During the workout, some cyclists took a swig of a liquid that contained glucose or maltodextrin, both carbohydrates. The cyclists did not swallow the drink but only swished it around in their mouth for 10 seconds before spitting it out. Another group of cyclists were given a third drink containing artificial sweeteners.

Those who rinsed their mouths with the glucose or maltodextrin concoctions had a 2- to 3-percent better workout than those who used the artificially sweetened water. Researchers also looked at the brain activity of the athletes by using a magnetic resonance imaging (MRI) machine. They found that the carbohydrate-laced drinks stimulated specific areas of the brain associated with pleasure or reward. Those who drank the flavored, sweetened water did not experience any additional brain function.

"Our results suggest that any carbohydrate in the mouth could improve exercise performance," Ed Chambers, a scientist who worked on the study, told WebMD.com. "However, this has only been demonstrated with glucose and maltodextrin and would need to be proven. We want to make clear that the study does not imply that athletes do not need to swallow energy drinks during exercise."

Q & A

Question: Will sports drinks improve my athletic performance?

Answer: Several studies have indicated that athletes performed just as well when drinking water as they did drinking a sports drink during an intense one-hour workout. However, for those who exercise for more than an hour, athletes have improved certain types of activities by consuming sports drinks rather than water.

LOWERING THE BAR

When Homer Simpson, the animated patriarch of TV's *The Simpsons,* decided to climb the "Murderhorn" to impress his son, Bart, he ate nothing but fictional Power Sauce bars. Homer thought Power Sauce, made of six different types of apples, could power him to the top of Springfield's highest mountain. Little did Homer know that the bars were really made from "apple cores and old Chinese newspapers."

The ingredients of the best-selling energy bars are not as bad as the Power Sauce bars, but nutritionists caution not to skip a balanced meal while using energy bars. Many of these bars are high in carbohydrates, which are found in other foods.

Researchers at Ball State University conducted a study on high-carb energy bars. They had nine cyclists ride for an hour to lower the level of stored glycogen in their muscles. The next day they rode their bikes for another half-hour and then sprinted. After resting for an hour, the researchers asked the cyclists to consume 1,000 calories in four hours by eating PowerBars, Tiger's Milk Bars, or cinnamon-raisin bagels. The cyclists then rode their bikes for another hour. Researchers the measured the athletes' energy output and sugar levels. The scientists found that those who ate the bagels had the same performance as those who ate the energy bars.

"The bagels resulted in the same aerobic performance as the energy bars," said researcher David Pearson, who was quoted in the *Nutrition Action Health Letter* published by the Center for Science in the Public Interest. "There's no magic to the bars. As long as you're getting the same number of calories and carbs in each food, there's no advantage to eating energy bars, and they're much more expensive." Moreover, Pearson said, the high-calorie, high-carb energy bars benefited only athletes who exercised for a long time. "People think, 'if top-grade athletes eat these bars, I need them for *my* workout.' That's a misconception," he said.

Some energy bars are high in protein. Nutritionists say you can get the same amount of protein from food. In addition, the amount of vitamins and minerals found in so-called supplement bars can easily be found in a vitamin pill.

See also: Calories and Weight; Carbohydrates and Exercise; Exercise and Strength; Sugar

FURTHER READING

KidsHealth.org. "The Buzz on Energy Foods." Available online. URL: http://kidshealth.org/teen/food_fitness/nutrition/energy.html#. Accessed June 2009.
Liebman, Bonnie, and David Schardt. "Bar Exam: Energy Bars Flunk." Center for Science in the Public Interest. Available online. URL: http://www.cspinet.org/nah/12_00/barexam.html. Accessed June 2009.

■ STEROIDS, ANABOLIC

Artificially manufactured chemicals derived from the male sex **hormone testosterone** and used to add body weight. The most common form of steroids is anabolic-androgenic. *Anabolic* steroids refer to muscle building, and *androgenic* refers to masculine traits.

Steroids can help an athlete become stronger. Athletes who use steroids can train harder for longer periods than athletes who do not abuse the drugs. In fact, many athletes in a wide range of sports have used, or are using, steroids to enhance their performance.

Barry Bonds, Alex Rodriquez, Roger Clemens, Marion Jones, and Kelli White are all phenomenal athletes, and all have been implicated in the use of steroids as performance-enhancing drugs. Athletes from body builders to baseball players have long used steroids to develop greater body mass and strength. In recent years, however, teenagers have been using these dangerous substances as they play college, high school, and middle school sports.

Some people, including nonathletes, abuse steroids to improve their physical appearance. Anabolic steroids can be taken either orally or by injection, usually in cycles of weeks or months, interrupted by shorter resting periods—a process known as *cycling.*

MEDICAL USE

Believe it or not, steroids were not manufactured to help athletes cheat. Long before athletes started using steroids, the drugs were actually prescribed for medical reasons.

The steroids that doctors prescribe the most are **cortisone** and other substances. Doctors use these drugs to treat a variety of ailments, including skin problems, rheumatoid **arthritis, asthma,** allergies, and a variety of diseases. Doctors also use steroids to treat a malfunctioning adrenal cortex, the part of the brain that regulates the body's response to stress. Steroids can also be used to treat delayed **puberty** in teenagers, some types of impotence, and the wasting of the body caused by HIV infection, the virus that causes AIDS.

ILLEGAL USE

People first became concerned about the illegal use of steroids in the 1970s, when the International Olympic Committee banned the use of the substances.

Since the beginning of athletic competition, athletes have tried various methods of cheating to gain the upper hand during competition. Even the ancient Greeks got in on the act. In ancient Greece, Olympians drank a beverage brewed from mushrooms and herbs to become stronger. The Romans chugged a specially made drink before competing in the Circus Maximus, where they raced chariots around a circular track.

The economics of sports is what fuels illegal steroid use. Many professional athletes say if they are not the best in their sport, they will not be offered the big-money contracts that are the staple of professional athletics. World-class athletes are not the only ones who use steroids. In 2002, a University of Michigan report stated that 4 percent of high school seniors and 3 percent of eighth graders used steroids.

Since that time, the issue of steroids has been discussed frequently in the media. Some teens are getting the message that illegal steroid use is bad for their health. Statistics provided by the National Institute on Drug Abuse show that the use of the drugs among eighth and 12th graders decreased in 2007. The survey discovered that roughly 2 percent of eighth, 10th, and 12th graders had taken anabolic steroids at least once in their lives. Those statistics showed a significant decrease from a 2002 study.

SIDE EFFECTS

The use of performance-enhancing drugs is known as "doping." While players may gain a slight advantage over their competitors by using steroids, the health risks associated with steroid abuse are putting many professionals and amateurs in danger. Anabolic steroids can damage the kidneys and liver and cause headaches, trembling, and cancer. Steroids can also wreak havoc on **hormones**. In men, steroid abuse can shrink testicles, reduce sperm count, and cause sterility. In women, steroid abuse can cause excessive facial hair growth and enlarged genitals and can also disrupt a woman's menstruation cycle. In short, women become more masculine. They grow more hair on their bodies, and their voices deepen.

Those who inject anabolic steroids and share the needles are at increased risk of developing various illnesses transmitted by body fluids, including HIV and hepatitis.

So-called roid rage is another problem associated with steroid abuse. A Northeastern University study found that steroids cause athletes to behave more aggressively long after they stop abusing the drugs.

In 2007, police found anabolic steroids in the home of professional wrestler Chris Benoit after he killed his wife and young son and hanged himself. Police suspected that steroid abuse played a role in the murders.

Q & A

Question: What are the signs of steroid abuse?

Answer: According to the Association of Steroid Abuse, there are many ways you can tell if someone is using steroids, although it might be difficult at times. Keep a watchful eye. Pay attention to the clothes the person wears and their hair. Any dramatic changes, such as a shaved head or a total overhaul of their wardrobe, are warning signs. Other signs include:

- Sudden muscle growth. If someone you know is getting unusually muscular, especially in the shoulders and neck region and across the chest and biceps, there is a good chance that they are abusing steroids.

- A significant outbreak of acne on the face or on the upper back and across the shoulders

- Mood swings or other shifts in behavior, such as being violent or combative

- Overuse of mouthwash or constant brushing of teeth. Steroid abusers often have bad breath.

- Paranoid behavior. Those who use steroids may become more secretive. They might hide their Internet searches.

A MAJOR-LEAGUE PROBLEM

While many sports have had incidents of athletes using performance-enhancing drugs, the problem seems to be most acute in professional baseball. Some of the game's biggest stars and role models have either admitted to using steroids or have been implicated in various steroid scandals.

The spotlight on steroids was focused on the sport in 2002, when federal agents raided the Bay Area Laboratory Co-Operative (BALCO) in Burlingame, California. At the time, agents seized various types of steroids and other chemicals from the lab. As a result, federal law enforcement officials ordered 40 athletes to testify about their relationship with BALCO and its founder, Victor Conte. Among those who testified were Barry Bonds of the San Francisco Giants and Jason Giambi, who was then the first baseman for the New York Yankees. On the heels of the BALCO investigation came word from Major League Baseball that more than 5 percent of the 1,438 players it tested for drugs took steroids.

Q & A

Question: Can someone be addicted to steroids?

Answer: It is possible that some steroid abusers might become addicted. Some may not care that their drug use is affecting their health and causing problems among family and friends. They also spend a lot of money to continue to use the drugs. Steroid abusers may also experience other symptoms associated with addiction, including mood swings, loss of appetite, reduced sex drive, and a desire to use more steroids. Many become depressed, even years after taking the drug.

From there, the steroid snowball began rolling downhill. Bonds, the all-time home run king, was implicated in the BALCO scandal. Despite his denials to the contrary, many people believe Bonds used performance-enhancing drugs. To find out how bad the steroid problem was in the game, Major League Baseball convened a blue ribbon commission to investigate steroid abuse. Dubbed the Mitchell Report after the committee's chairman, George Mitchell, Major League Baseball concluded that the use of performance-enhancing drugs had been pervasive in the sport for more than a decade.

One of the game's biggest stars, Roger Clemens, was named in the report, along with other players. Clemens denied the allegations. Then in 2009, New York Yankee slugger Alex Rodriguez admitted to using steroids when he played with the Texas Rangers.

See also: Exercise and Injuries; Exercise and Strength; Sleep and Physical Fitness

FURTHER READING

Aretha, David. *Steroids and Other Performance-Enhancing Drugs.* Berkeley Hills, N.J.: Enslow Publishing, 2005.

Lukas, Scott E. *Steroids* (Drug Library). Berkeley Hills, N.J.: Enslow Publishing, 2001.

Monroe, Judy. *Steroids, Sports and Body Image: The Risk of Performance-Enhancing Drugs* (Issues in Focus). Berkeley Hills, N.J.: Enslow Publishing 2001.

■ SUGAR

The simplest kind of carbohydrate, used by the body as a source of energy. Sugar is the generic term applied to several chemical compounds in the carbohydrate group that can be dissolved in water and are colorless, odorless, and have crystal structure. Sugars also are sweet to the taste. *Glucose, fructose,* and *galactose* are examples of the types of sugar in nature. Sugar is easily digested, a major source of energy in humans, and also used in cooking and baking.

Candies, cookies, cakes, and pies. What makes them sweet? Sugar. The average American consumes about two to three pounds of sugar each week. We put sugar in our coffee, in our cereal, and on our baked goods. Food manufacturers add sugar to their products.

When most people think of sugar, they think of table sugar, or *sucrose*, which comes from sugar cane and sugar beets. Sugar is a carbohydrate. In other words, sugar is formed when carbon, hydrogen, and oxygen atoms combine in various forms. A sugar's chemical composition determines how sweet the sugar is and how fast it dissolves in water.

Dextrose is another type of sugar, also called *glucose*, or grape sugar. *Lactose* is milk sugar, *maltrose* is malt sugar, and *fructose* is fruit sugar. Sugars are everywhere in nature. Fruits contain sugar. Vegetables contain sugar. Grains and seeds of plants also contain high amounts of starch, which can be chemically converted by an **enzyme** into simple sugars.

Plants make sugar via **photosynthesis**. Sugars are also found in the tissue of various animals. Simple sugars are called *monosaccharides*. The most abundant sugars in nature are hexose sugars, which are characterized by the presence of six carbon atoms in each **molecule**.

Of all the sugars, glucose is the largest and most complicated sugar molecule, also known as blood sugar. Fructose is the sweetest of the sugars and is found in fruit, honey, and high-fructose corn syrup, a product that food manufacturers use as an additive in products. Galactose is found in milk.

BLOOD SUGAR

Have you ever wondered what powers your body? What moves your legs? What moves your arms? What keeps your heart beating and your lungs breathing? Like any machine, the body needs fuel. That fuel comes in the form of glucose, or blood sugar. Every time you eat, your body converts carbohydrates to glucose.

Carbohydrates are chemical compounds containing carbon, hydrogen, and oxygen atoms. When you eat, your body's digestive system converts carbohydrates to glucose. Insulin, which is a hormone, helps the body process glucose, which your body turns into energy. Your body also stores some glucose in the liver and muscles and some as fat.

Hypoglycemia is a medical condition caused by too little sugar in the blood. Low blood sugar can cause fatigue, forgetfulness, and poor concentration.

A drop in blood sugar can impact your body's organs and systems. For example, glucose is the main nutrient that your nervous system needs to function properly.

Too much blood sugar in your blood causes **hyperglycemia.** Eating too much food is the main cause of the condition. Eating food that is high in sugar can also lead to elevated levels of glucose in the blood stream. Symptoms of hyperglycemia include frequent urination, dry mouth, weight loss, blurred vision, and excessive thirst. If your blood sugar level is high for an extended period, you are at risk of developing complications from diabetes, such as eye and kidney damage, along with heart disease.

The body also stores sugar in the form of **glycogen,** the source of energy that the body uses during exercise. Many athletes use glycogen during intense, short workouts. Glycogen also supplies energy during prolonged exercise, such as jogging. If there is not enough glycogen in a person's system during exercise, they quickly become fatigued, hindering their ability to continue to exercise or compete. The more carbs an athlete eats, the better they perform.

METABOLISM

Your body processes sugar by a process called **metabolism.** The body's digestive track breakdown carbohydrates, such as starch, into simple sugars containing six carbon atoms. Once broken down into simple sugars, the carbs can easily pass through the wall of the intestine. Fructose, however, does not have to be broken down, and can be fully absorbed by the intestines.

The body uses various enzymes, such as amylase, found in saliva and in the intestine, to digest carbohydrates. Other enzymes in the small intestines also breakdown carbs. The sugars pass through the wall of the small intestine and into blood vessels. Some sugar is stored in the liver as glycogen, which is available always to be converted to glucose.

HEALTH HAZARDS

While sugar is necessary for you to live, consuming too much sugar is not so sweet. Sugar can cause tooth decay, which occurs when the enamel on the outer surface of a tooth is destroyed. The destruction is caused by **bacteria** that collect on the tooth enamel. The bacteria live in a sticky, white film called plaque. The bacteria feed on sugar and create an acid that attacks the tooth enamel and causes it to rot.

Sugar has gotten a bad rap when it comes to diabetes. A person's intake of sugar does not cause diabetes. Diabetes occurs when the body's system that regulates blood sugar fails because of a lack of the hormone insulin. When that happens, glucose cannot pass into the body's cells to be used as energy. The glucose then builds up in the blood, leading to an abnormally high blood glucose level.

The response by your body to high levels of glucose can be devastating as it tries to eliminate excess sugar. Your body then has to use fat and proteins from your muscles for energy. When that happens, the body's natural process of converting glucose to energy is disrupted.

Sugar also contributes to obesity, although it is not the only cause. Eating more calories than you burn adds weight to the body. A tablespoon of sugar contains between 50 and 60 calories. A 12-ounce non-diet soft drink will have three tablespoons of sugar—totaling between 150 and 180 calories.

Fact Or Fiction?

Sugar is empty calories.

The Facts: Sugar does not provide any proteins, minerals, or vitamins to your body. In that respect, sugar provides no other nutritional benefit except fueling your body. Each gram of sugar has about four calories of energy.

Many nutritionists warn people to limit their intake of sugar. The World Health Organization says people should limit their sugar consumption to 10 percent of daily calories, while the National Academy of Sciences recommends limiting sugar intake to 25 percent. Research also links drinks high in sugar with *gout,* a painful disease of the joints. Sugar has also been blamed for hyperactivity in children, but a 2008 study in Britain claims there is no relationship between the two.

See also: Blood Sugar, Insulin, and Diabetes; Calories and Weight; Carbohydrates and Exercise; Dieting and Weight Loss; Nutritional Guidelines and Healthy Diets

FURTHER READING

Bennett, Connie, and Stephen Sinatra. *Sugar Shock! How Sweets and Simple Carbs Can Derail Your Life and How You Can Get Back on Track.* New York: Penguin Group, 2007.

Fittante, Ann. *The Sugar Solution Cookbook*. New York: Rodale, 2006.

■ VEGETARIANISM AND VEGANISM

The practice of excluding meat and animal by-products from a diet. There are several forms of vegetarianism, including veganism. Vegans, as they are often called, not only exclude all animal products from their diets but are also staunch supporters of animal rights. Vegans eat only food from plants. The definition of veganism is "a philosophy and way of living which seeks to exclude—as far as is possible and practical—all forms of exploitation of, and cruelty to, animals for food, clothing, or any other purpose."

To that end, vegans do not use toothpaste that contains calcium taken from animal bones. They also oppose the cruel treatment of animals in various industries, such as the meat and cosmetic industries.

There are varying degrees of vegetarianism. Most vegetarians do eat cheese and eggs, drink milk, and eat fish. Those who practice *lacto-vegetarianism* eat dairy products but exclude eggs. Those who practice *ovo-vegetarianism* eat eggs, but will not consume dairy products. Those who are *lacto-ovo vegetarians* eat both eggs and dairy products. *Semi-vegetarians* eat fish and poultry as well as dairy products and eggs.

VEGETARIAN DIETS

The reasons for following a vegetarian diet are many. Some people choose the diet because of moral convictions. They simply believe that humans should not eat animals. Others follow a vegetarian diet because of religious or cultural reasons. Many vegetarians, however, also think abstaining from meat is a healthier way to live.

Eating a vegetarian diet means keeping close tabs on nutrition. Vegetarians, especially teenage vegetarians, need to make sure they are getting enough protein, calcium, iron, zinc, and other nutrients to keep their bodies healthy. The less restrictive a vegetarian diet is, the easier it is to get the proper amount of nutrients into the body.

HEALTH BENEFITS

Since there are varying degrees of vegetarianism, it is difficult to adequately research the healthful effects of the various diets and to make a general statement about each of them. However, vegetarians tend to practice healthier habits. They generally maintain a healthy weight and do not abuse tobacco, illicit drugs, or alcohol. Moreover, they are physically active.

Their lifestyles also help vegetarians maintain a healthy blood pressure, and they also seem to have healthier hearts than nonvegetarians. Since diet is a major factor in heart disease, vegetarians fare better than meat-eaters. Heart disease is related to the consumption of **saturated fats** and **cholesterol**. In general, vegetarian diets are low in saturated fats and cholesterol. Vegetarian diets are also high in dietary fiber. Their **lipids,** fatty acids found in animal fats and oils, are also low.

DID YOU KNOW?

Vegetarian Diet Pyramid

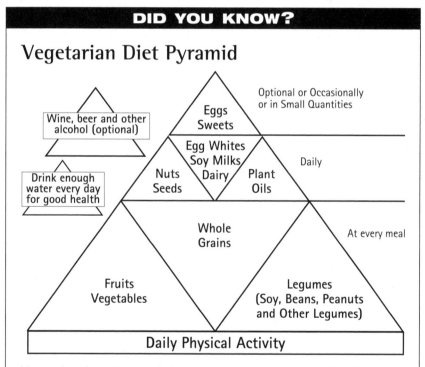

Wine, beer and other alcohol (optional)

Drink enough water every day for good health

Eggs
Sweets

Egg Whites
Soy Milks

Nuts
Seeds

Dairy

Plant
Oils

Whole
Grains

Fruits
Vegetables

Legumes
(Soy, Beans, Peanuts
and Other Legumes)

Optional or Occasionally
or in Small Quantities

Daily

At every meal

Daily Physical Activity

Vegetarians have their own food pyramid. The Vegetarian Diet Pyramid was developed in the 1990s by researchers from Cornell University and Harvard University. This pyramid stresses that a wide range of certain foods be eaten at every meal, particularly fruits and vegetables, whole grains, and legumes—such as peas and beans.

Source: Oldways Preservation & Exchange Trust, Cornell University,1998.

Studies show that when vegetarians are fed meat, their lipid levels worsen. When meat-eaters go on a vegetarian diet, their lipid levels improve. One study concluded that coronary artery disease can be reversed by eating a low-fat vegetarian diet, along with reducing stress, not smoking, and exercising.

One study also showed that those who have been on vegetarian diets for most of their lives have a reduced risk for breast cancer. The study, conducted by researchers at the London School of Hygiene and Tropical Medicine, studied women who had come to Great Britain from India and Pakistan.

The researchers looked at women who were Hindus because they were more likely to be lifelong vegetarians. They also studied Muslims who were mostly meat-eaters. Scientists found that those who ate a vegetarian diet for most of the lives were less likely to develop breast cancer. They not only ate less meat, they ate more vegetables than those who did eat meat.

Other studies have looked at the cancer rate of Seventh-Day Adventists, a religious group who, as a rule, eat a lacto-ovo-vegetarian diet. Those studies suggest that the mortality rate from cancer of the group was less than the rest of the population. Scientists surmise the low cancer rates might correspond directly to their vegetarian diets and say their eating a lot of vegetables and fruits reduced the group's risk of cancer. In addition, people who suffer from colon cancer tend to eat a lot of meat.

HEALTH RISKS

Eating an all-vegetarian diet does have certain health consequences if the diet is poorly planned. Vegetarians need to pay attention to their energy intake, and they also need to make sure they are getting the proper amount of nutrients from the foods they eat.

Poorly planned vegetarian diets can affect pregnant women, children, and those who are sick. Plant-based foods do not supply the body with enough energy compared to food from animals. Vegan diets do not provide enough energy for children who are growing. To compensate for the loss of such critical nutrients in the diet, nutritionists recommend that vegan children eat a lot of legumes and nuts. Vegan children are often smaller in weight and height than their meat-eating peers.

Other problems associated with a poorly-planned vegetarian diet include

- ▇ Osteoporosis. The lack of calcium in a vegetarian diet could result in bone loss.
- ▇ Rickets. A lack of vitamin D in children can foster this disease, which impacts bone growth.
- ▇ Anemia. Low iron in the blood causes anemia.
- ▇ Emaciation or slow growth. A lack of protein can impact the growth of infants and children.

VEGETARIAN LESSONS

You want to be healthier, but you refuse to give up pepperoni pizza or ham steak. The thought of snacking on grapes, oranges, and nuts does little to whet your appetite. Frankly, you do not want to be vegetarian, but you want to live a healthier life style. How can you do it?

It is a good idea to limit your meat intake to at most one meal a week. When you go out to eat with your friends, do not order a cheeseburger. Instead, have a meatless dish. If you do eat meat, nutritionists recommend treating the meat like a side dish. Reduce the portion size and eat more vegetables, salads, legumes, and whole grains.

See also: Dieting and Weight Loss; Fats; Food Groups; Food Pyramid; Nutritional Guidelines and Healthy Diets; Nutritional Supplements

FURTHER READING

Krizmanic, Judy, and Matthew Wawiorka (illustrator). *The Teen's Vegetarian Cookbook*. New York: Penguin Books, 1999.

Serafin, Kim. *Everything You Need to Know About Being a Vegetarian* (Need to Know Library). New York: Rosen Publishing, 1999.

▇ VITAMINS

Any of the 13 chemically unrelated **organic compounds** that the human body needs in small quantities to function. Many vitamins are *coenzymes,* which are small **molecules** that help the body's enzymes work properly. The body does not produce vitamins. Instead, a person must eat food containing vitamins. Most of the vitamins a person needs can be found by eating a balanced diet. Vitamin deficiencies can result in numerous health problems, including scurvy, which results from a lack of vitamin C.

VITAMINS EXPLAINED

Vitamins stimulate normal growth and stave off disease. There are two types of vitamins: *fat soluble* and *water soluble.*

When you consume fat-soluble vitamins, you body stores the nutrients for up to six months. When it is time for your body to use those vitamins, special protein transporters move the vitamins to where they are needed. Vitamins A, D, E, and K are fat-soluble vitamins. You can eat large quantities of fat-soluble vitamins every once in a while since they are stored in the body to meet its needs over time.

Vitamin A, for example, also known as retinol, helps the eyes adjust to changing light. Vitamin A also helps bones and teeth grow strong. The mouth, nose, throat, and lungs depend on vitamin A to keep them moist. Dairy products, fish, and liver, among other foods, all contain vitamin A. Vitamin A deficiency will cause teeth to develop badly and bones to grow more slowly. Too much vitamin A will cause skin to dry up and itch and also causes headaches, nausea, and loss of appetite.

Vitamin D helps the body use calcium and phosphorus efficiently and is important for strong bones. A lack of vitamin D causes rickets in growing children and a flattening of the skull. In adults, vitamin D deficiency weakens bones and muscles. It has also been linked to various diseases, including certain types of cancer and high blood pressure.

Unlike fat-soluble vitamins, water-soluble vitamins are not stored in the body. Instead, they travel quickly through the body via the bloodstream. What the body does not use is passed when a person urinates. Since these vitamins move fast, they need to be replenished continually. Vitamin C and the B vitamins are water soluble.

The B vitamins are necessary for the body to metabolize food. This group of vitamins also makes red blood cells, which carry oxygen throughout the body. Foods such as whole-grain bread, fish, seafood, chicken, and meats all contain B vitamins.

Vitamin C is important for keeping the body's tissues in good shape and also helps fight infections. Foods such as oranges, strawberries, tomatoes, and broccoli contain vitamin C.

Riboflavin, or vitamin B12, is necessary for normal bone growth and for the production of some **hormones** and red blood cells. Niacin

DID YOU KNOW?

How Fat-Soluble Vitamins Impact the Body

Vitamin	Common Food Sources	Impact on Body	Deficiency Symptoms	Overconsumption Symptoms
A (retinol) (provitamin A, such as beta carotene)	Liver, vitamin A milk and dairy products, butter, whole milk, cheese, egg yolks, carrots, leafy green vegetables, sweet potatoes, pumpkins, winter squash, apricots, cantaloupe	Helps to form skin and mucous membranes and keep them healthy, thus increasing resistance to infections; essential for night vision; promotes bones and tooth development. Beta carotene is an antioxidant and may protect against cancer.	Mild: night blindness, diarrhea, intestinal infections, impaired vision. Severe: inflammation of eyes; blindness in children	Mild: nausea, irritability, blurred vision. Severe: growth retardation, enlargement of liver and spleen, loss of hair, bone pain, increased pressure in skull, skin changes
D	Vitamin D fortified dairy products, fortified margarine, fish oils, egg yolks. Synthesized by sunlight action on skin	Promotes hardening of bones and teeth, increases the absorption of calcium	Severe: rickets in children; muscle and bone weakness weakness in adults	Mild: nausea, weight loss, irritability. Severe: mental and physical growth retardation, kidney damage, movement of

(continues)

DID YOU KNOW? (CONTINUED)

			calcium from bones into soft tissues.
E	Vegetable oil, margarine, butter, shortening, green and leafy vegetables, wheat germ, whole-grain products, nuts, egg yolks, liver	Protects vitamins A and C and fatty acids; prevents damage to cell membranes	Almost impossible to produce without starvation; possible anemia in low birth-weight infants.	Generally nontoxic under normal conditions. Severe: nausea, digestive tract disorders.
K	Dark green leafy vegetables, liver; also made by bacteria in the intestine	Helps blood to clot	Excessive bleeding	None reported

The chart lists all fat-soluble vitamins, how they work, and what happens when a person takes too much (overconsumption) and too little (deficiencies) of these vitamins.

Source: Colorado State University, 2008.

How Water–Soluble Vitamins Impact the Body

Vitamin	Common Food Sources	Impact on the body	Deficiency symptoms	Overconsumption symptoms
Vitamin C (ascorbic acid)	Citrus fruits, broccoli, strawberries, melons, green peppers, tomatoes, dark green vegetables, potatoes	Formation of collagen, a component of tissues, that helps hold them together; wound healing; maintaining blood vessels, bones, teeth; absorption of iron, calcium, folacin; production of brain hormones, immune factors; antioxidant	Bleeding gums; wounds don't heal; bruise easily; dry, rough skin; scurvy; sore joints and bones; increased infections	Nontoxic under normal conditions; diarrhea, bloating, cramps; increased incidence of kidney stones
Thiamin (vitamin B$_1$)	Pork, liver, whole grains, enriched grain products, peas, meats, legumes	Helps release energy from foods; promotes normal appetite; important in function of nervous system	Mental confusion; muscle weakness; wasting; edema; impaired growth; beriberi	None known

(continues)

DID YOU KNOW? (CONTINUED)

Riboflavin (vitamin B_2)	Liver, milk, dark green vegetables, whole and enriched grain products, eggs	Helps release energy from foods; promotes good vision, healthy skin	Cracks at corners of mouth; makes eyes sensitive to light	None known
Niacin (nicotinamide, nicotinic acid)	Liver, fish poultry, meats, peanuts, whole and enriched grain products	Energy production from foods; acids digestion, promotes normal appetite; promotes healthy skin, nerves	Skin disorders; diarrhea; weakness; mental confusion; irritability	Abnormal liver function; cramps; nausea; irritability
Vitamin B_6 (pyridoxine, pyridoxal, pyridoxamine)	Pork, meats, whole grains and cereals, legumes, green, leafy vegetables	Aids in protein metabolism, absorption; acids in red blood cell formation; helps body use fats	Skin disorders, dermatitis, cracks at corners of mouth; irritability; anemia; kidney stones; nausea; smooth tongue	None known

Folacin (folic acid)	Liver, kidney, dark green leafy vegetables, meats, fish, whole grains, fortified grains and cereals, legumes, citrus fruits	Aids in protein metabolism; promotes red blood cell formation; prevents birth defects of spine, brains; lowers coronary heart disease risk	Anemia; smooth tongue; diarrhea	May mask vitamin B_{12} deficiency (pernicious anemia)
Vitamin B_{12}	Found only in animal foods; meats, liver, kidney, fish, eggs, milk and milk products, oysters, shellfish	Aids in building of genetic material; aids in development of normal red blood cells; maintenance of nervous system	Pernicious anemia, anemia; neurological disorders; degeneration of nerves that may cause numbness, tingling in fingers and toes	None known

(continues)

DID YOU KNOW? (CONTINUED)

Pantothenic acid (B₅)	Liver, kidney, meats, egg yolks, whole grains, legumes; also made by intestinal bacteria	Involved in energy production; acids in formation of hormones	Uncommon due to availability in most foods; fatigue; nausea, abdominal cramps; difficulty sleeping	None known
Biotin (B₇)	Liver, kidney, egg yolks, milk, most fresh vegetables; also made by intestinal bacteria	Helps release energy from carbohydrates; aids in fat synthesis	Uncommon under normal circumstances; fatigue; loss of appetite, nausea, vomiting; depression; muscle pains; anemia	None known

The chart lists all water-soluble vitamins, how they impact the body, and what happens in cases of overconsumption and deficiencies of these vitamins.

Source: Colorado State University, 2008.

is another important water-soluble vitamin that plays a role in helping the body's cells generate energy from food.

Q & A

Question: Can Vitamin C cure the common cold?

Answer: Despite claims to the contrary, vitamin C does not cure the common cold. However, it may lessen some of the symptoms. Some research indicates that vitamin C reduces the amount of histamine in the blood. If you have ever had a cold, you probably have had a runny nose or nasal congestion. Elevated levels of histamine in the blood causes nasal congestion—that's why you take an antihistamine to breathe again. Vitamin C stops histamine from tormenting you and also protects the lungs by reducing respiratory infections.

Q & A

Question: What is a multivitamin?

Answer: Multivitamins are supplements a person can take to augment the vitamins and minerals found in his or her diet. Multivitamins are recommended for those who have dietary imbalances or other nutritional needs. However, you have to monitor the concentration of the vitamins you are ingesting. Consuming large quantities of various vitamins can pose severe health risks.

BOLD CLAIMS

Over the years, a number of myths have been bandied about concerning what vitamins can do in relationship to a person's health. There are many people who claim that vitamins can cure certain illnesses. In fact, vitamins cannot cure an illness unless that illness was caused by a lack of a particular vitamin.

See also: Nutritional Supplements; Sports Drinks and Energy Bars

FURTHER READING
Reavley, Nicola. *The New Encyclopedia of Vitamins, Minerals, Supplements, and Herbs: How They Are Best Used to Promote Health and Well Being.* New York: Bookman Press, 1998.

Smith, Pamela. *What You Must Know About Vitamins, Minerals, Herbs & More: Choosing the Nutrients That Are Right for You.* Garden City, N.J.: Square One Publishers, 2008.

■ WEIGHT TRAINING AND WEIGHT MANAGEMENT

A form of **anaerobic** exercise that uses strength and resistance training to manage weight gain and weight loss. While proper nutrition and diet are essential in the struggle to lose weight, lifting weights will not only cause you to lose weight, it will strengthen your body.

Strength training can raise **metabolism** and allow the body to burn more calories. The more muscle you have, the more calories you will burn.

Strength training exercises give you power, agility, and strength by working the body's muscles against extra weight, known as resistance. Because your body's muscles work harder than normal, resistance training increases the amount of muscle mass in your body.

WEIGHT WORKOUT

One way to build muscle strength is to participate in an exercise program that uses weights. There are generally two different types of weights: free weights and weight machines. Free weights include barbells, dumbbells, and hand weights. Free weights work specific groups of muscles at a time. Weight machines, however, let you work on one specific muscle during workouts. People tend to use a variety of free weights and weight machines when they train.

STRENGTH TO THE MAX

The body's muscles use their power to contract. When working out, your body's muscles work against the weights. The cells of the body react to the extra resistance by becoming larger and stronger, which allows your muscles to contract easier.

When building muscles, you have to use more resistance than your muscles are used to, a concept called *overload*. However, you should lift only enough weight to allow you to complete the desired number of repetitions for that particular exercise.

Another key to weight training is *progression*. Your muscles will build more mass as you slowly increase the amount of weight you are lifting and the intensity in which you are lifting. You can make changes on a daily, monthly, or weekly basis. You should also train to a specific goal, a concept called *specificity*. Choosing a variety of exercises and repetitions that target different muscles will allow you to lose weight. Resting and giving your body a chance to recover is important because it allows your muscles to grow and change.

How does weight training burn calories? Any move your body makes burns calories. Weight loss comes from using more calories than you take in. Weight training burns calories at a low level, but the more muscle you have, the more energy your body needs to function properly. As such, with stronger muscles your body burns more calories and fat, even while you rest. As you burn fat, your body becomes leaner.

Aerobic training, however, burns calories much more quickly. Nevertheless, you can burn more calories during strength training by doing such exercises as squats and lunges. Working out the larger muscle groups in the lower part of the body burns more calories than working out the upper body, especially if you minimize rest periods between exercises. In other words, do not spend a lot of time resting between sets of exercises. Move as quickly as you can to the next set. This will not only burn more calories but allow you to become stronger.

In addition, alternate your strength training exercises with brief periods of aerobic exercises. This will burn three times more calories than lifting weights along. Using the correct weight is important. The key is to use a weight that is heavy enough to tire the muscles out. Experts say you can gauge if the weight is heavy enough by doing a single set of 12 repetitions. If you are using the proper weight, you should just barely be able to finish the last rep. However, if you are a beginner, you need to ease into your weight training program to minimize the chance of any injury.

See also: Aerobic Exercise; Dieting and Weight Loss; Exercise and Injuries; Exercise and Strength

FURTHER READING
Delavier, Frederic. *Strength Training Anatomy.* Champaign, Ill.: Human Kinetics, 2005.
Gallagher, Tony. *Weight Training for Beginners.* New York: HarperCollins, 2003.

HOTLINES AND HELP SITES

American Heart Association
URL: http://www.americanheart.org
Phone: 1-800-AHA-USA (1-800-242-8721)
Mission: A national voluntary health agency whose mission is to reduce disability and death from cardiovascular diseases and stroke. It also aims to reduce coronary heart disease by 25 percent, reduce smoking by 25 percent, and reduce high blood pressure by 25 percent. The American Heart Association has also taken on the task of eliminating obesity and diabetes.
Programs: Offers public health education about lifestyle choices such as exercise and tobacco use. The American Heart Association spends its money on research and a variety of educational programs that benefit the general public.

U.S. Department of Health and Human Services (Anorexia Nervosa)
URL: http://www.4women.gov/FAQ/anorexia-nervosa.cfm
Phone: 1-800-944-9662
Mission: Established in 1991 within the U.S. Department of Health and Human Services, the National Women's Health Information Center provides reliable and current information on women's health, including information on anorexia nervosa.
Programs: A variety of programs and information on a wide range of women's health issues, including violence against women and information on HIV. The Women's Health Information Center also holds summits, campaigns, and meetings on such topics as minority women's health, breastfeeding, and other topics related to women.

Shapeup.org

URL: http://www.shapeup.org/atmstd/kitchen/faqtxt.html#2

Mission: Founded in 1994, Shape Up America is a not-for-profit organization dedicated to raising awareness about obesity and other health issues. Its goal is to provide good information on how to manage healthy weight.

Programs: The organization has a variety of programs to help individuals manage their weight, including interactive tools for health professionals to guide them in determining a patient's obesity-related health risks. Shapeup.org also includes information and interactive tools to help parents manage the weight of their children.

America Academy of Pediatrics (Sports Injuries)

URL: http://www.aap.org/advocacy/releases/sportsinjury.htm

Phone: 1-202-347-8600

Mission: The American Academy of Pediatrics is an organization of 60,000 pediatricians concerned with the health and well-being of children.

Programs: The academy provides many programs, publications, and activities with information on sports injuries, immunizations, Internet safety, and other childhood health topics. The AAP's main goal is to draw attention to the fact that most children in the United States do not get the health care they need.

National Institute of Arthritis and Musculoskeletal and Skin Diseases

URL: http://www.niams.nih.gov/

Phone: 1-877-22-NIAMS (877-226-4267)

Mission: Part of the National Institutes of Health, the National Institute of Arthritis and Musculoskeletal and Skin Diseases supports research into the causes, treatment, and prevention of various diseases of the muscles, skeleton, and skin. The organization also provides basic training for scientists to carry out research and provide information on these diseases.

Programs: The organization provides a number of programs including developing a supplemental health curriculum for students in sixth to eighth grades. "Looking Good, Feeling Good: From the Inside Out (Exploring Bone, Muscle, and Skin)" highlights NIAMS scientific research and provides students with an opportunity to understand how the skin, muscle, and bone systems contribute to health.

U.S. Department of Agriculture Center for Nutrition Policy and Promotion

URL: http://www.cnpp.usda.gov/default.htm

Phone: 1-703-305-7600

Mission: To improve the health and well-being of Americans by developing and promoting sound dietary guidance that corresponds with current scientific research into diets and health.

Programs: The USDA provides many programs including the MyPyramid Menu Planner, which outlines the basic dietary guidelines for eating a healthy diet and being physically active. The USDA is also responsible for the Food Pyramid. Its staff consists of nutritionists, nutrition scientists, economists, and policy experts.

President's Council on Physical Fitness and Sports

URL: http://www.fitness.gov

Phone: 1-202-690-9000

Mission: The President's Council on Physical Fitness and Sports is a committee of volunteers who advise the president of the United States on physical activity, fitness, and sports in the United States. The goal of the council is to promote health, physical activity, and fitness through participation in sports, especially among children.

Programs: In an effort to promote better health through physical fitness, the President's Council on Physical Fitness and Sports has developed the Presidential Challenge. The program is designed so a participant earns presidential awards for daily physical activity and fitness efforts.

U.S. Food and Drug Administration

URL: http://www.fda.gov/default.htm

Phone: 1-888-INFO-FDA (1-888-463-6322)

Mission: The U.S. Food and Drug Administration, or FDA, is an agency run by the U.S. Department of Health and Human Services. It consists of many offices. The chief function of the FDA is to protect the public health by assuring the safety and security of human and veterinary drugs, biological products, and medical devices. The FDA is also charged with making sure the food supply is safe. The

FDA regulates vaccines, cosmetics, radiation-emitting products, and tobacco, among others.

Programs: The FDA provides information on a variety of topics, including drug safety and licensed vaccines. It is also responsible for product recalls and safety alerts. Part of the FDA's wide-ranging responsibility is to encourage, build, and maintain cooperation around the world with other regulatory agencies to develop use standards and guidelines to safeguard and improve public health. The FDA also sponsors education, outreach, and technical programs.

National Cancer Institute

URL: http://www.cancer.gov

Phone: 1-800-4-CANCER (1-800-422-6237)

Mission: The National Cancer Institute is an agency run by the U.S. National Institutes of Health. Established under the National Cancer Institute Act of 1937, NCI is the principal agency in the United States for cancer research and training. Among other things, the NCI supports and coordinates research projects conducted by universities, hospitals, and research foundations. It also has its own laboratories.

Programs: The NCI has many programs related to cancer research and prevention. It works closely with volunteer organizations in cancer research and training activities and also provides information and statistics on cancer. It provides funding for hospitals, universities, and foundations. The institute also has a variety of advisory boards, including the President's Cancer Panel, which monitors the development and activities of the National Cancer Program, and the Cancer Advisory Board, which advises the secretary of the U.S. Department of Health and Human Services.

GLOSSARY

acute a sharp, sudden, and severe pain or reaction

aerobic how the body increases the flow of oxygen during physical activity

allergens foreign substances, such as pollen or ragweed, that cause an allergic reaction

amenorrhea the absence of three menstrual cycles

amino acid a small molecule that is one of the building blocks of protein and valuable in nutrition

anaerobic not requiring the release of oxygen during physical activity

anemia a blood disorder caused by a lack of iron in which there are too few red blood cells

antidepressants medications used to relieve the symptoms of depression

antioxidants substances that prevent cell damage from oxidation, keeping the fats and oils in foods from becoming rancid when exposed to air, thereby increasing the shelf life of certain foods; vitamins C and E are antioxidants

arteries vessels that carry blood from the heart to the rest of the body

arthritis inflammation of the joints with pain, swelling, and restricted motion

aseptic preventing infection

asthma a chronic lung ailment characterized by difficulty in breathing due to spasm of the air passages

atherosclerosis narrowing of coronary arteries due to the buildup of deposits in them

bacteria microscopic single-celled organisms that lack a nucleus and can cause disease

biopsy removal of living tissue from the body for diagnostic examination

body fat a normal part of the human body that stores energy as fat for metabolic demands

calories units of energy

carcinogens cancer-causing agents

cardiovascular pertaining to the heart and blood vessels

carpel tunnel syndrome a painful disorder of the hand caused by repetitive motion, such as typing

cartilage flexible tissue made up of the protein collagen

celluloses complex carbohydrates composed of long chains of glucose units and the principal units of the cell wall

Cesarean section the delivery of an infant by a surgical incision through the abdominal wall and uterus

cholesterol a soft, waxy substance present in all parts of the body, including the skin, muscles, liver, and intestines

chronic long-lasting or repeated

colorectal relating to the colon and rectum

compounds a substance that contains two or more atoms

compulsive obsessive, repetitive, ritualized

concussion an injury to the head that results in temporary unconsciousness

cortisone a steroid known for its anti-inflammatory qualities

dehydration the loss of water from the body

dementia the loss of intellectual ability as a result of the physical deterioration of brain cells

dentin a material that is harder than bone and makes up the bulk of a tooth

deoxyribonucleic acid (DNA) a complex, giant molecule that contains the chemically coded information needed for a cell to function

dioxin a carcinogenic compound used in industry

diuretics substance that increase the amount of urine excreted from the kidneys

dopamine a neurotransmitter found in the brain that helps transmit messages between brain cells

dwarfism a genetic condition that results in small stature

electrolyte ionized salts in the body, including sodium and potassium

emulsifiers   food additives that thicken

endocrine system   glands that control the body's metabolic activity

endorphins   natural substances produced by the pituitary gland and hypothalamus that regulate a variety of things, including reducing pain, regulating hunger, and the release of sex hormones

estrogen   female sex hormone

gastrointestinal tract   the organs that make up the digestive system

genes   the units of inherited material that determine the particular characteristics of an individual, such as height, weight, and eye and hair color

genetics   inherited characteristics passed down from generation to generation

glucose   a form of sugar that is present in the blood stream and provides the main source of fuel for the body

glycogen   a starch stored in the muscles that can be converted into glucose, which is stored in the liver and later used to generate energy

gums   complex carbohydrates formed by many plants and trees

hemoglobin   a protein in the blood that transports oxygen from the lungs to the rest of the body

histamines   substances released in damaged tissue that account for many of the symptoms of allergies

homogenize   to process by breaking up and dispersing the fat in milk so the cream will not rise

hormones   chemical substances produced by the endocrine system that control regular body functions

hyperglycemia   a physical disorder that results in abnormally high blood sugar

hypoglycemia   a physical disorder in which the body does not produce enough sugar, resulting in abnormally low blood sugar

hypothalamus   the region of the brain that regulates certain body functions, including water balance, temperature, and the production of the hormones in the pituitary gland

insulin   a hormone produced by the pancreas that regulates blood sugar, enabling cells to convert glucose to energy

iodine   an element that can improve the body's circulation system

isometric   involving muscular contractions against resistance without movement

lactose intolerant   being unable to metabolize lactose, a sugar found in milk

laxatives   drugs taken to increase bowel movements

ligament   band of tough tissue that connects bones to form moveable joints

lipids   any one of a group of fats or fatlike substances

lymph nodes   small masses of tissue found in the underarm, groin, neck, and abdomen that remove waste and fluids from the lymphatic system

lymphatic system   the network of tissues and organs that carries lymph (a clear, watery fluid containing proteins, salts, glucose, and other substances) throughout the body

malnutrition   a condition of poor nutrition that results from a poor diet

mast cells   cells that contain histamines that are involved in the production of inflammatory reactions associated with allergies

menopause   the cessation of a woman's reproductive ability

metabolism   occurring in the body's cells, the chemical activity in which those cells release energy from nutrients that allow the cells to grow and function

microorganisms   tiny organisms, such as bacteria or fungi, invisible to the human eye

molecules   groups of two or more atoms

mutations   changes in the genetic material of an organism, such as a cell

neurotransmitters   chemicals in the body that relay signals between cells

nitrates   additives used as preservatives and as coloring agents in cured meats, such as bacon and sausage

norepinephrine   a hormone and neurotransmitter secreted by the adrenal glands that governs the body's autonomic nervous system, especially blood pressure and heart rate; prepares the body for stress

organic   derived from nature

osteoporosis   a disease in which bone becomes brittle

pasteurization   the treatment of foods to reduce the number of microorganisms they contain to protect consumers from disease

pathologist   a scientist concerned with the study of disease processes and how they change the structure and function of the body

photosynthetic   relating to photosynthesis, the process by which plants turn radiant energy from the Sun into food

physiological   relating to the study of physiology, the study of living organisms

postmenopausal   after menopause

potassium   the main electrolyte in the body's cells, which, along with sodium, is important to the functioning of the nervous system

preservatives   food additives that stop food from spoiling

psychotherapist   a health professional who deals with mental and emotional disorders

psychotherapy   the treatment of psychological disorders

puberty   the time of life when the sex glands begin to function

relapses   setbacks

remission   the absence of a disease in patients with known chronic illnesses, such as cancer

salmonella   any groups of bacteria that cause food poisoning

saturated fats   fats that contain the fatty acid found in animal products, including cheese, milk, butter, and fatty meat

self-esteem   one's opinion of oneself

serotonin   a hormone and a neurotransmitter involved in sleep, depression, and memory

stress   emotional strain or discomfort felt from the pressures of life

stroke   the interruption of the blood supply to part of the brain due to a sudden bleed in the brain, known as cerebral hemorrhage

synthetic   substances that are human-made, or manufactured

tendon   a band of tissue that connects a muscle to a bone

testosterone   male sex hormone

toxic   poisonous

trans fats   a type of processed fat that does not occur in nature; usually used in baked goods such as donuts, breads, and potato chips

tumor   an abnormal mass of cells

unsaturated fats   fats that help to lower blood cholesterol if used in place of saturated fats; even unsaturated fats should be consumed in limited quantities because of their high calorie count; monounsaturated and polyunsaturated fats are two types of unsaturated fats

veins   blood vessels that carry blood toward the heart

INDEX

Boldface page numbers indicate extensive treatment of a topic.